25 Natural Ways to Lower Blood Pressure

JAMES SCALA, PH.D.

Keats Publishing

Chicago   New York   San Francisco   Lisbon   London   Madrid   Mexico City
Milan   New Delhi   San Juan   Seoul   Singapore   Sydney   Toronto

Library of Congress Cataloging-in-Publication Data

Scala, James, 1934–
     25 natural ways to lower blood pressure : a mind-body approach to
health and well being / by James Scala.
       p. cm.
     Includes bibliographical references and index.
     ISBN 0-658-00702-5 (alk. paper)
     1. Hypertension--Alternative treatment. 2. Hypertension--Popular works. 3. Mind
and body therapies--Popular works. I. Title: Twenty five natural ways to lower blood
pressure. II Title.
    RC685.H8 .S257 2001
    617.1'3206--dc21   2001029857

Keats Publishing

A Division of The McGraw·Hill Companies

3 4 5 6 7 8 9 0 DOC/DOC 0 9 8 7 6 5 4

ISBN 0-658-00702-5

This book was set in Garamond by Wendy Staroba Loreen
Printed and bound by R. R. Donnelley & Sons—Crawfordsville

Cover design by Mike Stromberg/The Great American Art Co.

This book is printed on acid-free paper.

Contents

Introduction

Over 25 percent of all adults and over 5 percent of people below age eighteen develop high blood pressure. When high blood pressure begins in adolescence, about 25 percent of its victims will have measurable heart damage by age eighteen. About 85 percent of all high blood pressure can be completely controlled by diet, food, and lifestyle.

Very few things we do have favorable results 85 percent of the time. For instance, investment and job decisions we make seldom meet our expectations. But if you follow the steps in this book carefully and consistently, you will have about an 85 percent probability of controlling your high blood pressure without resorting to medication.

You will also reap dividends in many other areas of health beyond just controlling blood pressure. Your risk of heart attack and stroke will diminish directly because high blood pressure increases risk of both. Similarly, the likelihood that you will develop serious heart irregularities, such as angina, will lessen. Other less obvious benefits include the reduced likelihood of kidney problems, adult-onset (Type 2) diabetes, and even some visual problems that result from high blood pressure. Because blood pressure control always involves weight control, you will be less likely to have joint problems as you age because excess weight worsens them.

In spite of those clear physiological benefits, the greatest benefit is psychological. You will have demonstrated to yourself and your loved ones your perseverance and willpower—your ability to face a health problem head on and defeat it. The increased self-esteem derived from that accomplishment is incalculable.

I am always amazed at how much we can control our health and our destiny. The steps in this book are easy compared to other challenges people take on as individuals. For example, obtaining an undergraduate degree, let alone a doctorate, takes more work and dedication than the twenty-five steps described in this book. Yet, over 93 percent of these people with advanced degrees who develop high blood pressure will simply take medication for their condition without attempting control through diet and lifestyle.

Ask yourself the following questions:

- Why not select foods that work for you and not against you?
- Why not choose a lifestyle that works for your benefit?
- Why not set an example for the next generation?

1

Understand High Blood Pressure

Gaining control of blood pressure begins with understanding what constitutes normal blood pressure and what is high blood pressure. Armed with this knowledge, you can take appropriate steps to bring your blood pressure back to normal.

THE MARVELOUS VASCULAR SYSTEM

The body is a marvelous system that is both complex and wonderfully simple. It consists of about fifteen trillion cells, which are grouped into tissues and organs. These organs are further organized into systems. Each cell, organ, and organ system has a specific purpose. The organs involved in blood pressure include the skin, heart, lungs, kidneys, and some glands. The systems involved are the cardiovascular and excretory systems. Most tissues, especially the muscle and vascular tissues, are also critically involved.

Each individual cell requires many nutrients, with oxygen being the most important. As nutrients are metabolized, waste products, the most abundant of which is carbon dioxide, accumulate and must be removed. The cardiovascular system, a specialized complex organ system, is responsible for the distribution of nutrients and the removal of wastes from each cell.

The heart pumps bright red, oxygen-laden blood into the largest artery, the aorta, which branches into smaller and smaller arteries called arterioles and capillaries. Arterioles and microscopic capillaries infiltrate every tissue, carrying oxygen and other nutrients to each cell. The venous system then carries waste-laden blood to the lungs to remove carbon dioxide and to the kidneys to remove other wastes. The cleansed blood returns to the heart and is then pumped out for another voyage through the system.

The arterioles and veins that bring blood to and from the muscles and skin constitute the *peripheral circulatory system.* Besides bringing nutrients to the cells and removing wastes, this system is essential in regulating body temperature. Peripheral blood flow regulates temperature by either increasing blood flow to the surface to radiate heat into the environment or restricting blood flow to conserve heat. During exercise, for example, blood flow is increased not only to meet nutrient demands of the tissues but also to radiate heat. Conversely, in a cold environment, blood flow to the surface is reduced to conserve body temperature.

Since the heart's job is to pump blood, it is easy to understand why pressure is essential. Like any other fluid pump, the heart pushes the blood around with a force we call blood pressure. Because the heart pushes the blood into the arterial system on a single stroke, two pressures are important: the systolic or higher pressure is the force generated when the blood is pushed into the arteries; the diastolic or lower pressure remains in the system when the heart's pumping chamber, the left ventricle, relaxes to fill again with blood as it gets ready for the next push.

Normal adult blood pressure, on average, is 120 systolic and 80 or less diastolic, simply expressed as 120 over 80. Individually, the numbers correspond to millimeters of mercury, but when expressed as a fraction, such as 120/80, the figures have no absolute value and are simply relative. Although blood pressure is no longer measured against a column of mercury measured in millimeters, a mercury column is used to calibrate the instruments, so the unit remains meaningful, and some physicians still use these devices.

Normal blood pressure is that of an average, healthy individual of a particular age group. It can vary rather widely; for example, my blood pressure is usually 110 over 70 or less, and sometimes it is as low as 100/60. On occasion, when I'm very nervous or active, it soars to 130/90. A rule of thumb teaches that systolic should be 100 plus your age, up to age twenty, and diastolic should be 40 less than systolic. So, for our purposes, normal is 120/80, and recognize that a little higher or lower is still within safe bounds.

HOW BLOOD PRESSURE DEVELOPS

Blood pressure is the amount of blood pumped, the rate of pumping, and the resistance that it must overcome. In medical terminology, we say that blood pressure is the product of cardiac output and total peripheral resistance. It follows that there are two major determinants of blood pressure: heart output and the factors that restrict blood flow.

Heart (Cardiac) Output

Cardiac output is the result of stroke volume, or the amount of blood expelled by each contraction of the pumping chamber, multiplied by the actual number of beats per minute.

Total Peripheral Resistance

Once blood is pumped from the heart, the resistance to flow is determined by three factors: the flowability or viscosity of the blood, the elasticity or flexibility of the venous and arterial systems, and the number and diameter of the arterioles.

Blood viscosity describes blood's ability to flow. Viscosity means the resistance of liquid to flow. For example, honey has a high viscosity; it doesn't flow easily. By contrast, water has a low viscosity. Blood with low viscosity flows more easily than that with high viscosity.

The elasticity of the arterial and veinal walls describes their ability to stretch. They can be like a set of rigid pipes or flexible and stretchable like a rubber hose that handles surges in water pressure by giving and relaxing. Neither the arterial nor the venous systems are meant to be rigid conduits. On the contrary, each should be flexible and capable of distending and contracting. The less rigid the arteries, the lower the blood pressure will be.

Likewise, by distending or contracting, the venous system becomes a dynamic reservoir that can determine how much blood from each stroke is returned to the heart. If the venous system is rigid and constricted, the return volume will be large. Consequently, each stroke must expel a large volume, which can elevate blood pressure because the heart has a larger task to perform.

Diameter and abundance of the arterioles is the third and usually the most dominant factor that determines blood pressure. The arterioles that bring blood to the muscles and skin make up the peripheral blood flow. The more dilated the arterioles and the more flexible the venous system, the lower the blood pressure will be.

Total peripheral resistance consists of the viscosity of the blood, the elasticity of the arteries and veins, and the number, size, and state of the arterioles. All three factors contribute to blood pressure. If viscosity is high, the arterial and venous systems are rigid, and arterioles are few and small, blood pressure will be higher. Therefore, by reducing blood viscosity, increasing the number and size of the arterioles, and causing arteries to relax, blood pressure can be reduced because the total peripheral resistance will be less. This can be accomplished by the effective use of exercise and lifestyle changes.

HOW HIGH IS TOO HIGH?

In 1913, a father-and-son team of physicians, the Janeways, reported that about 11 percent of their patients had systolic blood pressure over 165 millimeters of mercury. Significantly, they also noted that these patients didn't live as long as those whose systolic pressure was not so high. It is now accepted by all health agencies worldwide that the more elevated the blood pressure, the greater the risk of an early death from a variety of illnesses, ranging from heart attack and stroke to kidney failure. It's important to diagnose the presence of high blood pressure early and to deal with it effectively.

In 1984, the National Committee on High Blood Pressure published its conclusions in the Archives of Internal Medicine and established a classification system for blood pressure (see Table 1.1).

Table 1.1

Classification of Blood Pressure

Category of Hypertension	Range in Millimeters of Mercury Diastolic BP
Normal blood pressure	Less than 85
High normal	85 to 89
Mild hypertension	90 to 104
Moderate hypertension	105 to 114
Severe hypertension	115 or higher
	Systolic BP When Diastolic BP Is Less Than 90
Normal	Less than 140
Borderline isolated systolic hypertension	140 to 159
Isolated systolic hypertension	160 or more

Blood pressure doesn't go from normal to severe hypertension overnight; it creeps up slowly. Diastolic pressure over 80 millimeters of mercury is a warning sign that diet and lifestyle should change. Insurance companies consider high blood pressure when selling a life insurance policy, an indication of its seriousness.

Less than 10 percent of high blood pressure cases are the result of a specific problem, such as kidney disease, an adrenal tumor, or constriction of the major artery (the aorta). When such a cause is identified, this condition is called *secondary hypertension,* because it is the by-product of another illness. When that illness is corrected, the hypertension usually disappears.

Common high blood pressure, which accounts for over 90 percent of all high blood pressure cases, is called *essential hypertension.* It is usually the result of many factors combined, including heredity, excess weight, poor diet, and lack of fitness, to name the most common. This book deals with essential hypertension.

SYMPTOMS OF THE SILENT KILLER

High blood pressure is called the silent killer because many people with the problem never know they have it. Of the fifty million Americans with high blood pressure, only about thirty million have been diagnosed. The rest may never know until they go to a doctor for another reason—a physical for insurance purposes, a stroke, heart attack, kidney failure, or some other problem either caused by or having nothing to do with high blood pressure—and have their blood pressure taken in a workup.

If your diastolic blood pressure went from 70 one day to 105 the next, you'd immediately get symptoms. But blood pressure usually creeps up slowly, often over many years, and your body adjusts to the gradual change. You feel "normal" until that day your doctor or the nurse says, "Your blood pressure's too high!" However, you may experience the following symptoms, which can be early warning signs of high blood pressure.

- Headaches, especially in the morning
- Ringing in the ears
- Unexplained dizziness
- Spontaneous nosebleeds
- Depression without apparent cause
- Blurred vision
- Tension when there is no cause
- Flushing of the face
- Fainting spells

CAUSES OF HIGH BLOOD PRESSURE

Seldom is high blood pressure the result of only one problem. Indeed, most common high blood pressure is the outcome of many factors that have accumulated over the years. Following is a list of common causes.

- Alcohol
- Dietary fat imbalance
- Low dietary K-factor (sodium-potassium balance); excess sodium chloride (salt)
- Excess weight
- Heredity
- Insulin overload
- Poor nutrition
- Poor fitness
- Stress
- Type A personality traits

About 85 percent of all high blood pressure cases can be reversed by deliberate changes in diet and lifestyle. About two-thirds of the remaining 15 percent can significantly bring down their need for medication by the same measures. This means that nearly everyone with high blood pressure can dramatically lower his blood pressure by actions he takes. This book provides steps you can take to reduce if not cure high blood pressure.

Keep Score

Succeeding at anything requires keeping score; we all need a quantitative scale to chart our progress. The simplest health index most people use is climbing on the bathroom scale to chart weight loss, or measuring their waist. If you want to get your blood pressure into line, you've got to keep track of your progress and keep track of what that all-important pump, your heart, is doing!

START WITH YOUR PULSE

Measuring your pulse is easy. Your pulse can be taken in many places, but I recommend the wrist. You'll need a watch or clock with a second hand; don't use a stopwatch.

While sitting, place your arm on a table so your elbow is about as high as your heart. Later on when you get good at it, you might want to measure your pulse while standing, holding your arm up in the air, or after exercising to get a feeling for its range during a typical day.

Now find your pulse at your wrist. If you're right-handed, use your left hand on your right wrist, pressing with the first two or three fingers on the right side of the wrist with the palm up. Keep trying until you find a steady beat. When you can feel it consistently, time it for a full minute. (When you get good you can time it for ten seconds and multiply by six, but for the time being, count it for a full minute to be accurate.)

From chapter 1, we know that the peripheral pressure results from both the number of beats per minute and the volume of each surge of blood your heart pumps. This implies that a lower pulse rate when resting is consistent with lower blood pressure. Generally, it's that way with most people; however, there are limits. Generally, the pulse rate should be below 80 beats per minute, with an average of about 70. Most people seldom have a pulse rate below about 60 beats per minute. Well-conditioned athletes and a minority of others have a low pulse rate; for example, I once measured a runner whose resting rate was 40!

BE CONSISTENT

Many things, such as exercise, eating, drinking, tension, and anxiety, to name a few, can cause variations in your pulse. However, if you take your pulse and your blood pressure consistently at the same time, under the conditions described above (sitting with your elbow as high as your heart), you can establish your norm and use it to set your objectives.

CAN YOU REDUCE YOUR RESTING PULSE RATE?

In most cases, yes! It's done by improving your physical fitness—developing an exercise program, getting your weight into line, and improving your diet. Jogging both improves the muscle tone of your legs and the muscle tone of your cardiovascular system. Your heart is a muscle and your arteries and arterioles are lined with muscle cells. To improve the fitness of these muscles, they need to be exercised beyond the normal everyday level. As they become more fit, they don't have to work as hard to get all that blood moved around; consequently, as fitness improves, your resting pulse and blood pressure usually decline.

Exercise can be swimming, brisk walking, cycling, rowing, skating, skiing, and other activities, including skill sports like tennis, handball, and so on. I'll return to exercise in chapter 15, but for now, see it as the means to improve cardiovascular fitness as well as muscle tone.

A word of caution: If you're starting an exercise program for the first time, start slowly. Discuss your plans with your doctor to be sure that the program you select is ambitious enough to be effective but not dangerous for you. If you're out of shape, you didn't get that way in a day or two. To get into shape, you'll require more than a day or two; in fact, it will require a month or two.

People can lower their pulse and blood pressure by willpower alone through biofeedback (explained in chapter 24). Biofeedback enables you to monitor your pulse and blood pressure, which you can then, through conscious effort, lower. With practice, it can help reduce high blood pressure. Meditation is another form of mental conditioning that reduces pulse rate and blood pressure. Meditation is explained in chapter 24.

MEASURE YOUR OWN BLOOD PRESSURE

Measuring your own blood pressure has become convenient. You can do it on a coin-operated machine in some stores or purchase a device like the one your doctor uses or one of the new electronic, battery-operated devices. The device for measuring blood pressure is called a *sphygmomanometer.*

Measuring blood pressure is simple. You wrap a band (the cuff) around your arm and stop all blood flow. Then, just below the band, you listen with a stethoscope to an artery and slowly release the band. As the blood starts flowing, the left ventricle or the systolic pressure comes through (the high number). As the lower pressure comes through, the beats stop, and the second sound is steady; that's the background pressure or the diastolic pressure (the low number).

The cuff is hooked to a pressure-sensing device, which is activated by pumping up the cuff. In the doctor's office, mercury is used to measure pressure, but many newer electronic devices are calibrated against a standard column of mercury and are almost as accurate. The electronic sphygmomanometer has a sound-sensing device more sensitive and objective than the human ear, so there's no need for a stethoscope.

I suggest you purchase one of the newer battery-operated, electronic sphygmomanometers that give you your systolic and diastolic blood pressures and pulse rate in one reading. They are sold in most drugstores, some discount and health stores, through mail order catalogs, and over the Internet. The sphygmomanometer you purchase will have directions on its use. There are a few commonalities that apply to all of them.

- Wrap the cuff snugly but not tightly.
- Pump the pressure in the cuff sufficiently to stop blood flow; about 200 to 225 millimeters is enough. When you're back in shape, 150 will be plenty.
- Let the air drain from the cuff slowly and steadily. Many devices do this automatically.
- Do not take only one measurement; use several measurements.
- Always measure with your elbow resting on a table at about the level of your heart, or midchest.

The battery-operated devices don't always give consistent measurements when used repeatedly in succession due to current surges and charge buildup. Inaccurate readings can also result from low batteries. If you opt for this type, be sure the batteries are good and always allow a few minutes between measurements.

If you're a purist, you may purchase the mechanical type, which requires a stethoscope to read the column of mercury. Once you become adept at using the stethoscope, your readings will be more accurate than those of battery-operated devices. You only need to learn how to listen for the blood flow at two different pressures: The first one is a beat-beat-beat and the second a steady flow. Keep practicing and you will get it correct. If you have trouble, ask a nurse or your doctor to show you.

The more you know and understand about your body, the greater respect you'll have for it, and the better care you'll take of it. To quote Satchel Paige as an old man, "Boy, if I'd aknown I'd need this body so long, I'd ataken better care of it."

It's crucial to monitor your blood pressure daily whether you do it or you have someone else do it, such as a nurse where you work, or a friend. The one measurement taken at the doctor's office every six or twelve months, when you're nervous or even anxious, is inadequate, and it's not practical to go to her office daily, let alone once weekly. Besides the impracticality, studies have shown that when a doctor takes a patient's blood pressure, it's generally on the high side. This problem even has a name, *white-coat hypertension.*

If you seriously want to control your blood pressure without drugs, you should measure progress daily, or at the very least every three days. And you should keep the data you accumulate on yourself in a diary. Blood pressure measured regularly and consistently is a quantitative picture of how your vascular system is working and the wear and tear it is receiving. It is more quantitative and more precise than most other measurements, such as weight, cholesterol, blood sugar, and so on. And the beauty of taking your blood pressure is that you can do it yourself quickly and gain an intimate knowledge of the inner workings of your body. But there's more. As you make progress in gaining control, you'll begin to see how much you control your own health. You'll realize that small changes in diet, a moderate amount of exercise, and a diversion or hobby can have a profound influence on your health. And you will realize that you are more in control of your health than you ever thought.

3

Establish a Family History

Every aspect of health has a hereditary component. Who our parents are influences our personality and behavior and the probability of our developing diseases, such as cancer. So what about high blood pressure? Until the recent decade, we had thought that high blood pressure was largely an inherited trait. After all, it was easy to identify families in which a significant percentage of family members in each generation had high blood pressure.

In support of the hereditary factor, Lewis Dahl, a scientist, bred laboratory animals with high blood pressure, proving that it can reside in our genes. However, careful research has now proven that it is not simply a case of having high blood pressure–prone parents.

The majority of some populations never develop essential hypertension or common high blood pressure. (About 1 or 2 percent in any population develops secondary hypertension due to illness; when the illness clears up, the blood pressure returns to normal.) We could erroneously assume those people are inherently resistant to high blood pressure, but if we follow people who emigrate from those societies into our society, about one-third of them will develop essential hypertension. Therefore, we can conclude that there is an inherited susceptibility in some people, and the disease is triggered by something in the environment. Alcoholism is similar; the tendency is there in some people just waiting for the right circumstances, such as stress or depression.

With blood pressure, the environmental factors are food, lifestyle, and stress. After all, we control the environment inside our body with food and drink. In the case of essential hypertension, our cardiovascular system becomes what we eat.

Food and lifestyle go together. Excess calories usually lead to excess weight, and excess weight leads to poor exercise habits. A lack of exercise doesn't dissipate the effects of stress, so they add to the growing problem. Undissipated stress also leads to food and often alcohol abuse to relieve stress, which contributes to overweight and an imbalance in the dietary sodium-potassium ratio. All these environmental factors heaped on the wrong genetic background can send blood pressure soaring.

Although you can't change your genetic composition, knowing where you stand is essential to how you approach diet, lifestyle, and personality. To have a better understanding of your task, you must conduct a family assessment to find out if you're the first with high blood pressure or just one more in a long family history. If you go through the genetic analysis in this chapter and conclude that you have an above average genetic risk, common sense indicates that you should take your high blood pressure very seriously and resolve to gain control.

HOW DO I KNOW IF IT'S IN MY GENES?

Doing a family high blood pressure history is the only way to determine your general genetic risk. It is not difficult, takes little time, and can be very interesting. All you have to do is construct a family tree going back a generation or two. If possible, write the age at which a relative was diagnosed and two other facts about them: Were they overweight? Did they exercise regularly? For an example, look at the sample family history in Table 3.1.

Table 3.1

Blood Pressure History of Gene's Family

Relatives	Blood Pressure	Weight
Siblings (and Self)		
Brother (older)	H	OW
Brother (younger)	H	N
Sister (younger)	N	N
Self (Gene)	H	N
Percentage of high blood pressure	75% (3 out of 4)	
Maternal Side		
Grandmother	N	NA
Grandfather	H	NA
Great uncle	H	N
Great uncle	N	N
Great aunt	N	N
Mother	H	N
Aunt	N	N
Uncle	N	N
Uncle	N	N
Male cousin	N	N
Male cousin	N	N
Female cousin	N	N
Female cousin	N	N
Percentage of high blood pressure	23% (3 out of 13)	
Paternal Side		
Grandmother	H	NA
Grandfather	H	NA
Great uncle	H	N
Great uncle	N	N
Great aunt	H	N
Father	N	N
Aunt	H	N
Uncle	N	OW
Uncle	N	N

Table 3.1 (continued)

Blood Pressure History of Gene's Family

Relatives	Blood Pressure	Weight
Paternal Side (continued)		
Uncle	N	N
Male cousin	H	N
Male cousin	N	N
Male cousin	N	N
Female cousin	H	N
Female cousin	H	N
Percentage of *high blood pressure*	53% (8 out of 15)	

Key: H (high), N (normal), OW (overweight)

In reviewing Gene's family, it appears that in recent generations about 30 percent of the family members have experienced high blood pressure. In a society where about 25 percent of men develop high blood pressure, Gene's family has a greater than average risk. You can construct a similar family tree in an afternoon by making some phone calls and sending some e-mails. Blood pressure is generally not something people are reluctant to discuss.

Look over Gene's family tree and make a few inferences. Although there aren't enough people in his family to draw hard conclusions, the history suggests the tendency is on his father's side. Another factor is weight: high blood pressure consistently shows up among overweight members. Again, a single family sample, though small, can be useful.

It is clear that not everyone in Gene's family gets high blood pressure. This suggests that the genetic link is not strong. Indeed, it gives

Gene a bright outlook and suggests that if he takes his health seriously, he'll probably be able to control his blood pressure by diet and lifestyle.

Suppose every male in Gene's family had high blood pressure. That consistency would indicate he has a harder, but not impossible, task. It might, however, be that he would never gain complete control and would always need medication.

WHAT TO LOOK FOR

In your own chart, look for patterns that suggest a cause for concern:

- Consistency. Is there a repeating pattern? A repeating pattern would be that over 30 percent in each generation developed high blood pressure, going through both parents and all grandparents, uncles, aunts, and cousins. Ideally, you could trace back to great grandparents, great uncles, and possibly even their siblings. Search for patterns of several men or women in each family with high blood pressure.
- Excess weight and physical fitness. Does a pattern of obesity show up? How about fitness? Do people who stay fit get high blood pressure?
- Alcohol. Do heavy drinkers in the family get high blood pressure?

Does heredity mean you are fated to have high blood pressure? Absolutely not! Unequivocally, heredity is not even an excuse any longer. In high blood pressure, the hereditary tendency is not a firm trait like eye color. It is simply a warning flag that says, "Take care of your body and everything will be just fine." I like to put it in a more positive way: If you've inherited the tendency, you're lucky because you know the boundary lines within which you must live. No need for you to experiment and search; you're in control of your health!

4

Understand and Take Care of Your Kidneys

We have two kidneys, each one about the size of an average adult fist, located in the abdomen just under the back muscles. Although we can function well on one kidney, our built-in excess capacity of two suggests kidneys are critical organs; nature supplies two to ensure survival.

The kidneys process and clear about 50 gallons of fluid daily. Within each kidney there are millions of specialized cells called *nephrons.* Each nephron is a marvelous filtering unit. Millions of nephrons working together make a filtering system with incredible capacity. The kidneys' ability to filter sodium and chloride from the blood and regulate fluid levels is one of the three systems of blood pressure regulation in the body.

Kidneys influence blood pressure by regulating fluid volume, including blood, and controlling the amount of sodium, potassium, calcium, and magnesium in our system. Because these minerals profoundly influence the state of tension or relaxation of the muscles in the arterioles, the kidneys affect peripheral resistance.

Blood passes through the kidneys, wastes are removed, and the remaining materials, including water, are returned to the bloodstream.

Waste products and the liquid that contains them are the urine we void. Most of the sodium and water that are removed get reabsorbed from the nephrons and returned to the blood. If there's an excess of sodium and fluid volume, the kidney cannot eliminate it. Blood pressure is elevated to overcome this situation and literally force the sodium out. This process is analogous to reverse osmosis used to purify water. If sodium didn't get reabsorbed, the problem of high blood pressure wouldn't exist.

SODIUM REABSORPTION AND DIET

Sodium gets reabsorbed as sodium chloride, or common table salt. Sodium reabsorption illustrates the body's excellent ability to conserve nutrients. This ability probably evolved as a mechanism to conserve sodium and chloride. Salt was so scarce just 2,000 years ago that it was a medium of exchange. In the Roman Empire, soldiers were paid with a salt ration. (The word *salary* comes from the Latin word for salt: *sal.*) In a few isolated areas, salt cakes are still a medium of barter.

In our modern world, salt is no longer rare and our excess consumption of those two once-rare elements works against us. Only in the last 1,000 years has salt become readily available. And only in the last 400 years has it become cheap. In the evolutionary process, 100,000 years is a "blink of the eye," let alone 2,000. In short, humanity's the same, and our kidneys are the same as they were 10,000 years ago, but the availability of salt has changed.

Reabsorption of sodium as sodium chloride can work against us by precipitating diet-related high blood pressure. Most processed foods contain large quantities of salt, and people often liberally add salt to food. Sodium and chloride as they occur naturally in unprocessed foods are probably not a serious problem. Unprocessed foods contain sodium in a myriad of forms, including very small amounts of sodium chloride. For example, sodium is found as citrate in citrus fruits and glutamate in grains. As a result, fruits, vegetables, and whole grains contain naturally balanced forms of sodium and don't have an excess of either sodium or chloride. In fact, the amount of chloride naturally present in foods, along with the body's ability to reabsorb 99 percent of sodium, suggests that very little dietary sodium is required. Normal active adults get along well on only about 300 milligrams of sodium daily, and some experts claim even less is sufficient.

Processed foods contain salt either as a preservative or to increase taste intensity. Return to natural foods, fruits, grains, vegetables, meat, fish, poultry—anything that grows from the ground, on the ground, on trees, walks, swims, or flies. Do not prepare or eat anything with elaborate sauces or coatings. Boil, broil, barbecue, bake, or poach without adding salt. It works! Unsalted food may seem bland at first, but in a short time you'll start savoring flavors that you didn't know were present. A new world of taste will open up to you. (See more on controlling salt in the diet in chapters 5 and 6.)

HORMONAL INFLUENCES

A number of hormonal systems influence the kidneys. All these systems when not functioning properly or in synchrony can cause sodium reabsorption, but they can be influenced by diet or drugs.

Excess insulin causes sodium reabsorption by the kidneys, indirectly elevating blood pressure. This makes people who produce excess insulin candidates for high blood pressure. Consequently, many overweight people, people who habitually consume excess sugar, and some diabetics who do not control insulin correctly develop high blood pressure.

Another more elaborate hormone system that influences blood pressure is the *angiotensin-renin-aldosterone system*. This system includes the adrenal glands that produce *aldosterone*, the primary hormone that induces the kidneys to retain sodium and chloride and excrete potassium. Aldosterone is produced by the two adrenal glands situated on top of each kidney.

Aldosterone causes the kidneys and the sweat glands (which act somewhat like kidneys) to retain sodium. Although aldosterone is produced by the adrenal glands, it is, in part, regulated by the kidneys. This regulation involves the hormone *angiotensin* and the enzyme *renin.*

Kidneys release renin, an enzyme that causes the release of another hormone, angiotensin. Angiotensin causes constriction of the arterioles and this signals the adrenals to release more aldosterone. Constriction of the arterioles and the release of aldosterone elevates blood pressure by two mechanisms: Arteriole constriction causes increased peripheral resistance, and aldosterone causes salt retention.

Stimulation of the sympathetic nervous system produces renin. This is the nervous system that takes charge when we're under stress. If someone attacks you, your kidneys release renin, and the entire angiotensin-aldosterone process is started. This takes our blood pressure discussion into the realm of stress, which we'll discuss in chapter 16.

Some physicians who specialize in hypertension talk of *high-renin producers.* High-renin producers are people, often with Type A personalities (see chapter 17), who normally produce excess renin. Excess renin leads to elevated blood pressure. In some cases, the only recourse is to control renin levels with drugs that block its production. Some evidence suggests that inadequate magnesium can cause excessive renin production.

Some serious conditions can also cause excessive aldosterone. These serious illnesses must be dealt with by modern medical intervention. In these cases, the high blood pressure is secondary to the illness (secondary hypertension) and cannot be dealt with by diet.

There are other factors not as well understood that influence the rate of sodium excretion by the kidneys. These materials, called *natriuretic factors* (meaning sodium-excretion factors), are produced in other parts of the body and influence how the kidneys handle sodium. Natriuretic factors are produced in response to increased blood sodium levels; therefore, diets high or low in sodium will influence their levels proportionately.

5

Balance Potassium and Sodium

High blood pressure results from many factors, but there's always one common denominator: excessive salt and an incorrect balance between sodium and potassium. You must understand these two minerals.

Potassium and sodium are the body's two major electrolytes, nutrients essential for nerve conduction, energy production, cell integrity, and many other functions of the body. Both conduct electricity. Salt, sodium chloride, dissolves to form the electrolytes sodium and chloride. Pure distilled water does not conduct electricity, but water containing salt does because sodium and chloride are ions, each containing an electric charge.

Each body cell in every tissue and organ is composed of and bathed in fluid. The fluid both inside and outside the cell contains many materials; most important among them are sodium, potassium, calcium, magnesium, and chloride. The intracellular fluid contains more potassium than sodium, so potassium is the predominant electrolyte inside the cell. Conversely, the fluid bathing the cell contains more sodium than potassium, so sodium is the predominant electrolyte in the extracellular fluid. Chloride complements both electrolytes. A deficiency of either sodium or potassium is generally not an issue because we can get all we need from food. However, most people get far too much sodium from food.

Having the correct balance of potassium and sodium, or *K-factor,* enables cells to carry out their functions. For example, cells that line the stomach must produce acid and digestive enzymes to break down food. The production of these essential factors requires energy. If those cells don't have the correct potassium-sodium balance, they can't produce those factors. Nerve impulse conduction, which causes you to pull your hand from a hot stove and "tells" your heart to beat, also requires the right ratio of sodium and potassium to function properly. The ratio of potassium to sodium in our body is critical, and when it becomes seriously distorted, the consequences can be life threatening. Inadequate dietary potassium, often resulting from fad diets, has been implicated many times in heart attacks.

Your body maintains a ratio of about three parts potassium to one part sodium. This ratio facilitates all the many functions that each cell must perform. This ratio is not unique to humans and is found throughout the animal kingdom. In contrast, a much higher ratio of potassium to sodium is found in the plant kingdom, 10 to 20 or more parts potassium to one part sodium. Plants don't have, among other things, a nervous system and the need to transmit nerve impulses and so require less sodium. This characteristic of plants is to our benefit; making vegetables a substantial part of your diet can help balance excess sodium.

Suppose the extracellular fluids become oversupplied with sodium. How does the body return things to normal? Initially, the body uses the kidneys to excrete excess sodium. But suppose the kidneys don't extract and excrete sufficient sodium from the blood? The peripheral vascular system then constricts and increases resistance to blood flow, causing the blood pressure to increase, which forces the kidneys to excrete more sodium. Elevation of blood pressure to eliminate more sodium shouldn't surprise anyone with engineering knowledge. Engineers do it all the time with a process called *reverse osmosis.* In reverse osmosis, pressure is elevated to force impurities across a membrane. Some home water purifiers use this method to make pure, mineral-free water. Unfortunately, when the body uses this process, blood pressure can increase to a dangerous level.

Constriction of the peripheral vascular system also causes the body to retain more fluid, which dilutes the extracellular sodium. If the fluid around a cell has a high concentration of sodium, simply increasing fluid volume dilutes the sodium, lowering the ratio of sodium chloride to potassium. Increasing fluid also enables the kidneys to excrete both water and sodium. The only problem is that the blood pressure is elevated to accomplish the task.

Normally these two mechanisms, reverse osmosis and fluid retention, work together to return the K-factor ratio to normal. If this elevation takes place often enough, however, the blood volume increases and the vascular system adapts and keeps the blood pressure elevated.

The medical profession first used diuretics to control high blood pressure. Diuretics cause the body to excrete more fluid and, with the fluid, sodium chloride. This method usually reduces blood pressure in its early stages. One major drawback is that diuretics also cause the kidneys to excrete potassium, so along with diuretics, doctors often prescribe potassium supplements. The person taking them must also drink more water. People who can correct high blood pressure with diuretics can easily solve their problem with diet. Indeed, if a diuretic works for you, control by diet alone is a certainty.

Unequivocally, diet has a profound effect on the sodium-potassium balance. Excess sodium comes from the food we eat; similarly, inadequate potassium is primarily a dietary shortfall. Around 1974, papers started appearing in medical journals indicating when the dietary potassium to sodium ratio, the K-factor, falls below 3 and drops to about 1 or even 1.5, high blood pressure increases dramatically. African Americans are especially vulnerable to high blood pressure because of how their kidneys handle chloride. Diabetic children are also likely to get high blood pressure. This research leaves no doubt that the dietary potassium to sodium ratio is critical and clearly indicates that the individual can control her blood pressure through the food she eats.

Natural foods, particularly vegetables, contain much more potassium than sodium. Indeed, the ratio in animal-derived foods (meat, fish, and poultry) of between 3 and 6 is low compared to vegetables, where the ratio is usually 10 or much more. Anthropologists estimate that the potassium to sodium ratio in the diet of our remote ancestors of 10,000 years ago was about 16! Their diet was much higher in potassium than in sodium, with a K-factor of 3 or more. In contrast, people in many developed countries, such as the United States, the United Kingdom, and continental Europe, now eat a diet in which the K-factor is about 0.8. The body must work overtime to excrete the excess sodium and retain potassium, which the body often accomplishes by, unfortunately, raising blood pressure.

Although the ratio of potassium to sodium is probably more important than the absolute amount of either, the average adult requires a minimum of about 200 or 250 milligrams of sodium daily. That translates to 650 milligrams of salt, while the requirement for potassium is about 1,000 milligrams. Some people cannot tolerate excessive sodium (above about 1,000 milligrams daily) even if their dietary K-factor is above 2 because they develop high blood pressure. Those numbers are minimum levels for maintaining good health, and they tell an important story: We require a lot more potassium than sodium.

The Food and Nutrition Board describes a safe and adequate range as 1,100 to 3,300 milligrams of sodium and 1,875 to 5,625 milligrams of potassium. Safe and adequate does not mean required. It means that most people who do not have high blood pressure can consume sodium in that range and remain in satisfactory health.

But to the government, satisfactory health means "free from overt symptoms," and they established these numbers before we understood the K-factor. It is important to note that most high blood pressure goes undetected.

Some experts have proposed that the government rewrite its recommendations, proposing an upper limit of about 1,500 milligrams of sodium and a K-factor of at least 3, which means about 4,500 milligrams of potassium. For people whose diastolic blood pressure has reached 85, their sodium limit should be reduced to 1,000 milligrams with a K-factor of 4 or more. No matter what numbers you use, the K-factor should be at least 3. When I look at the K-factor that occurs naturally in plants, with its high ratio of potassium, I conclude that the dietary K-factor should probably be greater than 4, perhaps as high as 10.

DIETARY CHANGES

Lay the groundwork now for your new dietary plan. One important part should be obvious: increase the potassium and decrease the sodium in your diet. Nature will do this if you give her a chance. Unprocessed foods, especially vegetables, are naturally high in potassium and low in sodium. In contrast, many man-made, highly processed foods are exactly the opposite: high in sodium and low in potassium (see Table 5.1). Therefore, most of these changes should be obvious.

1. Eat one to three fresh vegetables of any type at every meal except breakfast. These include leafy vegetables (lettuce, spinach), squash, tubers (potatoes), broccoli, carrots, plus a variety of other vegetables. Always boil, steam, or stir-fry; never add salt.
2. Eat whole grains and legumes (peas, beans), except black beans.

Table 5.1

K-Factor in Some Common Foods

Food	Sodium (mg)	Potassium (mg)	K-Factor
Apple	1	159	159.00
Avocado	21	1,097	52.00
Hot dog	461	71	0.15
Cornflakes	351	26	0.07
Roast beef (slice)	46	547	12.00
Corn	4	226	56.00
Apple pie (frozen)	298	73	0.24
Frozen meat loaf (5 oz.)	951	196	0.20

3. Start each day with a cereal that has more potassium than sodium. Some examples include oatmeal made without salt, Nabisco Shredded Wheat Bran Buds, puffed rice, wheat germ, and Quaker 100% Natural. Always use low-fat or skim milk, or a soy beverage.
4. Avoid processed foods that list salt as an ingredient. If you don't read the ingredients, now is the time to start!
5. Don't eat any processed food that doesn't clearly have the potassium and sodium content declared on the label. The potassium must be at least two times the sodium.
6. Don't eat any processed meat products, including poultry. Turkey or chicken bologna and similar products are still high in sodium.
7. Do not use salt on any foods. This will be tough, but you can do it. Alternatives are a hot pepper sauce such as Tabasco, horseradish, or salt substitutes. Herbs, spices, onions, and garlic go well with meat. Mrs. Dash's nonsalt herbs and spices are excellent.

8. For dessert, eat fresh fruit whenever possible. You can also eat ice cream, ice milk, and sherbet but avoid baked goods, pies, or cakes.
9. Purchase a low-sodium cookbook. Start using it for recipes.
10. Carefully read chapter 12 on dining out.

Some of these changes might be contrary to the way you have been eating, taken together, but they are a first, giant step toward reducing your blood pressure. More than that, once they become a habit, you will be on your way to optimizing your health.

6

Reduce Sodium

Supermarkets have some low-sodium foods available, and more are appearing all the time. You can help increase these foods by voting with money every time you purchase them because money counts to the manufacturer and the supermarket owner.

Low-sodium salad dressings are an outstanding example of food technology capabilities. For example, most brands of Russian or Thousand Island salad dressings provide about 125 to 130 milligrams of sodium per tablespoon (and who only uses a tablespoon?) and very little potassium, so their K-factor is nil. In contrast, low-sodium (and usually low-calorie) salad dressings contain only 2 milligrams sodium and 32 of potassium, giving them a K-factor of 16. Salads are already naturally high in potassium and low in sodium. By using one of these salad dressings, you make the salad still better and improve the flavor.

Other low-sodium foods, especially prepared foods like soup, seem bland because we are accustomed to more salt, but they can be spiced up. For example, a single drop of Tabasco adds only 2.5 milligrams of salt (an insignificant amount), and six drops can make a low-sodium soup taste much better, at a cost of only 15 milligrams of sodium. Or try adding a tablespoon or less of horseradish. Horseradish adds 17 milligrams of sodium and 52 milligrams of potassium, improves the K-factor, and adds a modest amount of texture.

SALT SUBSTITUTES

In general, the best salt substitutes are not made from potassium chloride. Remember, sodium retention is really salt retention. If you get sodium from one source and chloride from another, the nephrons in your kidneys can't distinguish them; they sense only sodium chloride, or salt. Therefore, you must read the label carefully and select products made from other potassium salts. Potassium gluconate and potassium bitartrate are the most common.

Salt substitutes can improve a meal with their potassium content. There are times when they serve as more than a flavor enhancer in cooking and are necessary to the recipe, such as in low-sodium bread. In addition, other people eating with you will appreciate the flavor they add to the food. Salt substitutes are excellent for those occasions but should be used only when necessary.

Salt substitutes are good for cooking but not essential, and they can lead to overconsumption of potassium. While 5,000 to 10,000 milligrams (5 to 10 grams) of potassium should be fine, it is possible through excessive use of salt substitutes to exceed that level. More than 10 grams of potassium is excessive, so use salt substitutes cautiously and emphasize spices and herbs instead.

The best salt substitutes are not substitutes at all; they are seasonings made from herbs and spices. Two excellent ones can be found on your supermarket's condiment shelf: Vegit All Purpose Seasoning and Mrs. Dash All Natural Seasoning.

SAUCES AND GRAVIES

Most commercial sauces and gravies are not acceptable on this dietary plan. They are prepared with far too much salt, and there is no room for compromise. There are some available that provide taste without salt, but you must search them out. Nature can solve your taste problem with garlic, onions, shallots, spices, and other herbs. For example, a little garlic sautéed in olive oil on a barbecued or broiled steak, hamburgers, fish, or poultry is an excellent seasoning. Try grated ginger over fish, poultry, and salads or sautéed with other foods to accomplish the same objective—good taste and good health.

FOOD TABLES: DO'S AND DON'TS

Table 6.1, at the end of the chapter, will help you select foods that will give you a new lease on life. Serving size is usually expressed as 3.5 ounces (100 grams) or as a single piece of fruit or other convenient serving.

Cooked Cereals

Do's

Cooked cereals are excellent if no salt is added in their preparation. Instant cooked cereals (add hot water) are often unacceptable because salt is used in the processing. Milk is not included in these servings; it is tabulated separately. Each cup of milk or soy beverage adds 120 milligrams sodium and 375 milligrams potassium.

Don'ts

Following the recipe on the box and adding salt destroys cooked cereal for this plan. These cereals taste excellent without added salt. If your taste buds crave salt, add six drops of Tabasco per serving. I know it sounds strange in cereal, but the taste is fine, and six drops adds only 15 milligrams. As another alternative, don't use milk; try your cereal with canned apricot nectar. It tastes great, reduces sodium, and elevates potassium even more.

Ready-to-Eat Cereals

Do's

Milk is not included in these servings; it is tabulated separately. A cup of milk usually adds 120 milligrams sodium and 375 milligrams potassium to each serving. See milk tabulation where low sodium is expressed, however.

Occasionally

These cereals are borderline because, though they are moderate in sodium, they are not high in potassium. Consequently, they have a poor K-factor. The addition of milk elevates the sodium content very close to the 200-milligram cutoff even though the K-factor is acceptable. Therefore, use them only occasionally and remember to eat other low-sodium, high-potassium foods in compensation.

Don'ts

Most ready-to-eat cereals cannot be used on this plan. I have identified those that can be served. Those that have sodium on the nutritional label should be avoided.

Milk for Cereals and Beverages

Do's

All milk, whether canned, dry, condensed, or whole, are do's for beverages or for cereals. The sodium in milk is not in the form of sodium chloride (salt), and although it is higher than desirable, it is acceptable. Low-sodium milk is available. I strongly recommend avoiding high-fat milk and using the low-fat varieties.

Beverage Mixes for Milk

Milk mixes are fine, but be sure to add the sodium and potassium from the milk to the total figures. Chocolate powder, a common mix for milk, contains, on average, 54 milligrams sodium and 168 milligrams potassium for a K-factor of 3.

Eggs

Do's

In general, eggs are acceptable because the sodium is not in the form of sodium chloride and their protein quality is excellent.

Don'ts

Though eggs are acceptable on this eating plan, the method of preparation can cause trouble. If you fry, don't add salt to the oil. Omelets should be made with a few drops of Tabasco or horseradish in place of salt. They should always be vegetarian, with ingredients such as onions, mushrooms, and tomatoes.

Breads

Do's

Oroweat bread is the most readily available low-sodium bread. Two slices of this bread contain only 10 milligrams of sodium. Available in the frozen section, it thaws quickly and can be used for toast or for sandwiches. Its sodium content is insignificant.

Don'ts

Breads and baked goods account for much of the hidden 5 to 10 grams of salt that Americans consume daily. If you like sandwiches and want to beat high blood pressure, you must learn to like Oroweat or other low-sodium bread. Not all grocers carry Oroweat bread, but other brands are available; usually in the frozen section. Be sure to ask.

Fruit

Do's

Fruit toppings for cereals and fruit as an accompaniment to any meal, especially breakfast, is excellent. Fruit is not only acceptable, it is highly recommended. You can't eat too much fruit, nor can you eat too many varieties. Note that in the table I have tabulated the average value; please be aware that sizes vary, as well as varieties of fruit.

Fruit Juices

Do's

Fruit juices, like fruit, are generally low in sodium and rich in potassium. They can be used to offset a meal component that is not rich in potassium but is low in sodium. For example, a poached egg on Oroweat toast and a glass of apple juice are balanced in sodium and potassium, even though the egg itself is not. Except where noted, serving size is 8 ounces.

Don'ts

Any fresh fruit and fresh fruit juice is excellent on this plan. Therefore, the only don'ts are sugary processed juice drinks that contain only a small amount of real juice. Fruit is not canned or frozen with salt, so it is usually fine; similarly for fruit juice. You can't use too much of either category.

Meat

Most nonorgan meats are fine. Chapter 8 will help you reduce the fat content and consequently your caloric intake. I have included the percentage of calories from fat for beef, pork, and white meat and broken it into low-, medium-, and high-fat selections, listing the high-fat meat for occasional consumption. Low-fat meat, in general, is excellent on this diet. It is low in sodium, rich in potassium, and if lean cuts are selected with excess fat trimmed, its caloric content is fine.

How meat is prepared, including poultry, is important. In general, poultry is excellent for any dietary program. If it is roasted, broiled, or barbecued without skin, or the skin is removed after cooking, it is low in fat and excellent in sodium and potassium, but even poultry can be high in fat if not selected correctly. Meat should always be broiled or barbecued without sauces or salt. Condiments, such as garlic, onions, shallots, ginger, and other herbs and spices, add flavor and zest to meat without increasing either its fat or sodium content. In the meat section of the table, serving size is the standard 3.5 ounces.

Do's

In general, low-fat cuts of meat provide less than 25 percent of their calories as fat. Medium-fat cuts provide 26 to 40 percent of their calories as fat. Both low- and medium-fat cuts are acceptable on a weight-controlled diet.

Occasionally

These cuts of meat are fine for control of high blood pressure, but because of their high fat content, they are recommended only occasionally and never on a weight-loss diet. Over 40 percent of their calories are derived from fat.

Organ meats, listed on page 54, are usually excessive in fat, but I have selected a few that are moderate in fat. Some organ meats are so high in sodium that, even though it is not always sodium chloride, it is often excessive for our purposes.

Don'ts

Virtually no processed meats can be eaten by people following this plan to control high blood pressure. Processed meat, whether beef, veal, lamb, or chicken and turkey ersatz meats, such as turkey pastrami, bologna, and franks, is simply unacceptable. Since these foods are unacceptable, I have not included sodium, potassium, or the K-factor ratio.

Beef to Avoid

- Beef burgundy
- Breakfast strips
- Corned beef
- Frozen meatloaf
- Frozen or canned chipped beef (several brands)
- Frozen or canned salisbury steak
- Frozen or canned sliced beef

Pork to Avoid

- Bacon bits
- Canadian bacon
- Cured bacon
- Cured ham
- Ham loaf
- Ham steaks
- Sausages (including bockwurst, blood, bratwurst, Polish luncheon, smoked, and turkey)
- Sweet and sour pork

Veal to Avoid

- Frozen veal parmigiana

Luncheon Meats, Franks, and Spreads to Avoid

- Barbecue loaf
- Bologna of all types
- Corned beef loaf
- Frankfurter
- Loaves (olive, mother's, pepper, pickle, picnic)
- Mortadella

- Salami of all types
- Sandwich spreads
- Turkey ham, turkey loaf, pastrami
- Vienna sausage
- Seafood

Seafood

Do's

In general, fish contain fat that is polyunsaturated, and many fish are low in fat. There is a sodium concern, however, because many fish contain over 75 milligrams in a normal serving. Although this is a caution, it is minor, since the sodium is usually not in the form of sodium chloride (salt). Therefore, select fish at least two or three times weekly, and use shellfish in moderation.

Fish is best when baked, broiled, or poached. If you fry it, do so without added salt and in olive oil. For zest and flavor, use ground ginger, bay seasoning, and other spices and onions, garlic, and shallots. A few drops of Tabasco are excellent.

Occasionally

Shellfish must be eaten with caution in this dietary program. Although low in fat, it is often high in sodium. Exceptions are soft clams and oysters. One serving of shellfish can use up 25 percent of the daily allowance of 800 milligrams of sodium; therefore, menu planning is absolutely critical when these fish are used.

Don'ts

Don't use processed, breaded, or batter-dipped fish, especially fish fillets. This list does not include sodium and potassium content because these foods are too high in sodium to be acceptable under any circumstances. Low-sodium processed fish is available, however, which is acceptable on this dietary plan.

- Crab cakes, deviled crab, or crab imperial
- Crab, canned
- Fillet almondine
- Fish fillets or other pieces, breaded and seasoned
- Fish, canned or packed in brine, unless specified as low sodium
- Fish sticks, breaded and frozen
- Lobster Newburg
- Lobster paste
- Oysters, clams, or mussels, canned or frozen
- Sardines in any sauce
- Shrimp, breaded, french fried, or as a paste

Vegetables and Legumes

Do's

Fresh and frozen vegetables are excellent for this dietary plan. They are naturally high in potassium and low in sodium. Do not use frozen mixed vegetables, however, unless they are on the do list of prepared mixed frozen vegetables. And, never, under any circumstances, use canned vegetables. Likewise, avoid canned beans and use dried. Soaking and cooking beans from scratch is time consuming but enables you to eliminate salt in their preparation.

Vegetables can be prepared in a variety of ways, ranging from boiling to frying in a wok with small amounts of oil. None of these methods will change their sodium-potassium content. However, when cooking vegetables or starches such as potatoes, rice, low sodium pasta, and so on, never add salt.

Snacks

Do's

The word *snack* is often synonymous with highly salted or sugary foods eaten between meals, such as chips, fries, and doughnuts. But snacks can be apples and vegetables, such as carrot sticks. These foods, with their excellent potassium content, actually have a beneficial effect on high blood pressure. The table lists acceptable snacks if no salt is added.

Don'ts

All other processed snacks are unacceptable unless you can purchase snacks that have no sodium added or provide less than 25 milligrams sodium in a normal serving.

Beverages

Do's

An average adult (150 pounds) requires 64 ounces of water daily. Most is obtained from a variety of beverages ranging from coffee to beer. However, people with high blood pressure should strive to drink six 8-ounce glasses of water daily. Make sure the water is low in sodium. Charged seltzer water into which gas is injected is fine. However, bottled soda water usually contains sodium.

Occasionally

Many carbonated beverages contain more than 75 milligrams of sodium, with insufficient potassium to redeem them. Therefore, they do not appear in the table. In contrast, some beverages do appear because their sodium content is low enough that their overall contribution is insignificant if used in moderation and if the diet is correct.

Desserts

Do's

Desserts are often an important part of the meal, and dairy products provide an excellent opportunity for eating pleasure without penalty. Whenever possible, whether you're eating ice cream or sherbet, top it with any fresh fruit. The fruit not only provides variety and eating pleasure but also contributes potassium without a sodium penalty.

Some puddings and gelatin desserts are borderline, but if served with fruit, or whipped topping, the sodium-potassium K-factor ratio is acceptable. Some, like gelatin desserts, are fine, especially when fruit is added to the mix or served as a topping. Your store may carry another brand. If so, it probably has a composition similar to the ones shown here.

A variety of dessert toppings are acceptable. For some people cream is essential in coffee, on fruit, or as a whipped cream topping on desserts. The products listed in the table can effectively convert fruit from a low-sodium snack to a great dessert. You gain the low sodium and high potassium of fruit with the taste and texture of whipped cream.

Occasionally

I do not advocate the use of candy; it is something we can do without. However, it sometimes seems unavoidable. Remember our discussions about excessive insulin!

Salad Dressings and Condiments

Do's

Low-sodium products are excellent for this plan. Other condiments such as Tabasco sauce can also be used to make plain, low-sodium food taste much better.

Don'ts

Mustard and Ketchup

Neither of these condiments is acceptable on this program. Learn to use other flavorings.

Soups

Do's

Low-sodium soups generally taste bland and seem watery, but they can be made much better with the addition of four to six drops of Tabasco or a tablespoon of horseradish. Low-sodium onion soup, tomato, or cream of mushroom are all excellent if made more tasty as suggested.

Don'ts

Canned soups are unacceptable. Dry soups are even worse. For example, a serving of many of these soups provides over one gram of sodium, all in the form of sodium chloride. I have not listed these products because they are simply too high in sodium and their potassium content is even worse. Do not be coerced by the statements "no salt added" or "homemade"; the sodium content is still excessive.

Spices, Herbs, and Flavorings

Do's

For thousands of years, spices and herbs have been used to enhance the flavor of foods. Spices were also used to protect food from spoiling and to hide the taste of bad food. We are no longer faced with problems of contaminated or spoiled food. We now use herbs, spices, and condiments strictly for pleasure. In this way they help us to eat foods without salt and rich in potassium. All amounts are one teaspoon.

In the amount of one teaspoon, the sodium content in most herbs and spices is trace or equivalent only to 1 milligram. Potassium is 20 to 30 milligrams, making the K-factor 20 to 30.

Don'ts

You cannot use flavored salts. These are mostly salt, flavored with other ingredients.

Oils

Do's

Cooking Oils

Polyunsaturated fatty acids, such as sunflower and safflower oils, should not be used for frying or sautéing because heating these oils to high temperatures can often change the natural structure from one that is safe and healthful to one that several studies have implicated in cancer. With both that and the need to prevent heart disease in mind, I have listed oils that I recommend in descending order of quality.

- Olive oil
- Peanut oil
- Sesame oil
- Shortening
- Soft margarine
- Butter

Oils for Dressing

For salad dressings or wherever oil is required in nonfrying cooking, I recommend light oils, high in polyunsaturated fatty acid (PUFA). The following list presents preferred oils, in descending order of quality.

- Safflower oil
- Sunflower oil
- Canola oil
- Corn oil
- Soybean oil

- Olive oil
- Peanut oil

Exotic Oils

Some gourmet stores provide oils from nuts that are especially rich in the omega-3 fatty acids that, in your body, produce eicosapentaenoic acid (EPA), such as walnut oil and almond oil.

Table 6.1 is not exhaustive. There are many low-sodium cookbooks and other books and resources available that provide food compositions listing sodium and potassium. In general, natural foods are fine so long as you don't add salt during their preparation. Frozen foods with no salt in the ingredients list are also fine.

Table 6.1		
K-Factor in Foods		
Sodium (mg)	Potassium (mg)	K-Factor
Cereals		
Cooked (serving size: 1 ounce)		
Barley 1 to 4	45 to 127	45
Corn grits, regular 0	54	54
Maypo 6	158	26
Oats 1	99	99
Ralston 3	115	38
Roman Meal 2	227	113
Whole wheat 1	129	129
Wheatena 4	140	35
Cream of Wheat 2	33	16
Ready-to-eat (serving size: 1 ounce)		
Frosted Mini Wheats 8	97	12
Granola Nature Valley 3	142	47
Puffed Rice 0	10	10

Table 6.1 *(continued)*

Cereals *(continued)*

	Sodium (mg)	Potassium (mg)	K-Factor
Ready-to-eat (serving size: 1 ounce) *(continued)*			
Puffed Wheat	1	50	50
Quaker 100% Natural	12	140	12
with raisins	12	139	12
with apples	14	140	10
Shredded Wheat and Shredded Wheat 'N Fiber	3	102	34
Wheat germ, toasted	1	268	268
C. W. Post with raisins	49	58	1.2
Heartland Natural	72	95	1.3
Heartland with coconut	57	104	1.8
Heartland with raisins	58	107	1.8

Dairy Products

	Sodium (mg)	Potassium (mg)	K-Factor
Milk (serving size: 8 ounces or 1 cup)			
Low-fat (1% fat)	123	381	3.0
Low-fat (2% fat)	122	377	3.0
Skim	126	406	3.2
Whole (3.5% fat)	122	351	2.9
Low-sodium whole	6	617	102.0
Skim dry (reconstituted)	161	538	3.3
Whole dry (reconstituted)	119	426	3.6
Eggs			
Eggs, 1 large	69	65	0.95
Omelet, 2 eggs (with ¼ cup peppers, ¼ cup mushrooms, ¼ cup onion)	150	271	1.8

Fruit

	Sodium (mg)	Potassium (mg)	K-Factor
Fresh, Canned and Frozen			
Apple, 1 medium (with skin)	1	159	159
Applesauce, canned (3½ oz. unsweetened)	2	91	45
Apricots, raw, 3 medium	1	313	313
canned	3	139	46
Banana, 1 medium	1	451	451
Blackberries, ½ cup (similar for canned and frozen)	0	141	141
Blueberries, 1 cup	9	129	14
Boysenberries, 1 cup, canned	2	207	104
Cantaloupe, 1 cup pieces	14	494	35
Cherries, 10 sweet	0	152	152
Cherries, 1 cup sour, canned	9	119	13
Dates, 10 dried	2	541	270
Figs, 1 medium	1	116	116
Fruit cocktail, ½ cup, canned	4	118	29
Grapefruit, ½ medium	0	158	158
Grapes, 1 cup	2	176	88
Honeydew melon, ¼ small	12	251	21
Kiwi fruit, 1 medium	4	252	63
Lemon or lime, 1 medium	1	80	80
Mango, 1 medium	4	322	81
Nectarine, 1 medium	0	288	288
Orange, 1 medium	1	250	250
Papaya, 1 medium	8	780	98
Peach, 1 medium, raw	0	171	171
canned, 1 cup	11	317	29
Pear, 1 medium	1	208	208
Pineapple, 1 cup	1	175	175
Plum, 1 medium	0	113	113

Table 6.1 *(continued)*

Fruit *(continued)*

	Sodium (mg)	Potassium (mg)	K-Factor
Fresh, Canned, and Frozen *(continued)*			
Prunes, 10	3	626	209
Raisins, ⅔ cup	12	746	62
Raspberries, 1 cup	0	187	187
Strawberries, 1 cup	2	247	123
Tangerine, 1 medium	1	132	132
Juices (serving size: 8 ounces)			
Apple juice	7	296	42
Apricot nectar	9	286	32
Cranberry juice	10	61	6
Grape juice	7	334	48
Grapefruit juice	2	400	200
Lemon or lime juice, 1 tablespoon	0	19	19
Orange juice	2	496	298
Papaya nectar	14	78	6
Peach nectar	17	101	6
Pineapple juice	2	334	167
Prune juice	11	706	64
Tangerine juice	2	440	220
Tomato juice or V-8 Juice (low sodium)	47	550	12

Meat

Beef			
Low-Fat Cuts			
Hamburger (lean)	41	480	11
Shank (lean)	60	370	6
Top round	46	547	12

	Sodium (mg)	Potassium (mg)	K-Factor
Beef *(continued)*			
Medium-Fat Cuts			
Bottom round	51	552	11
Chuck (selected lean)	60	370	6
Club steak (lean)	27	236	9
Flank steak	67	344	5
Porterhouse (lean)	26	232	9
Pot roast (lean)	18	152	8
Rib roast (lean)	17	169	10
Sirloin (lean)	34	349	10
High-Fat Cuts			
Chuck	60	370	6
Hamburger (medium fat)	40	382	9
Rib roast (lean and marbled)	57	438	8
Rib eye steak	60	370	6
Pot roast (lean and marbled)	43	309	7
Sirloin (lean and marbled)	57	545	9
Roast or ground T-bone	49	378	7
Tenderloin	30	288	9
Lamb			
Medium-Fat Cuts			
Arm chop (lean)	49	286	6
Leg (lean)	52	312	6
Leg (marbled)	82	492	6
Rib chop (lean)	43	252	6

Table 6.1 *(continued)*

Meat *(continued)*

	Sodium (mg)	Potassium (mg)	K-Factor
Lamb *(continued)*			
High-Fat Cuts			
Arm chop (marbled)	66	388	6
Blade chop (lean)	46	276	6
Loin chop (marbled)	37	218	6
Rib chop (marbled)	68	398	6
Pork			
Medium-Fat Cuts			
Blade (lean)	44	311	7
Butt (lean)	29	209	7
Ham fresh (lean)	54	382	7
Loin chop (lean)	41	386	9
High-Fat Cuts			
Blade (marbled)	78	551	7
Ham fresh (marbled)	61	434	7
Loin chop (marbled)	52	500	10
Tenderloin (lean)	55	509	9
Veal			
Medium-Fat Cuts			
Arm steak (lean)	46	452	10
Loin chop (lean)	47	342	7
Rib chop (lean)	35	329	9
Sirloin (lean)	38	342	9
Sirloin (marbled)	38	342	9

	Sodium (mg)	Potassium (mg)	K-Factor
Veal (continued)			
High-Fat Cuts			
Arm steak (marbled)	51	503	10
Chuck (medium fat)	80	500	6
Cutlet	54	527	10
Loin chop	54	384	7
Rib roast	80	500	6
Rib chop	41	387	9
Poultry			
Chicken			
Low-Fat Cuts			
Breast, roasted (without skin)	63	220	3.5
Drumstick, roasted (without skin)	42	108	2.5
Medium-Fat Cuts			
Breast (with skin)	69	240	3.5
Drumstick (with skin)	47	119	2.5
High-Fat Cuts			
Wing, roasted	25	57	2.0
Turkey			
Low-Fat Cuts			
Light meat, roasted (without skin)	64	305	4.8

Table 6.1 *(continued)*

Poultry *(continued)*

	Sodium (mg)	Potassium (mg)	K-Factor
Turkey *(continued)*			
Medium-Fat Cuts			
Dark meat (with skin)	76	274	3.6
Dark meat (without skin)	79	290	3.7
Ground turkey	74	260	3.5
Light meat (with skin)	63	285	4.5

Other Poultry

	Sodium (mg)	Potassium (mg)	K-Factor
Low-Fat Cuts			
Pheasant (without skin)	37	262	7.0
High-Fat Cuts			
Duck (with skin)	59	204	3.5
Duck (without skin)	65	252	3.9
Goose (with skin)	70	329	4.7
Goose (without skin)	76	388	5.0

Organ Meat

	Sodium (mg)	Potassium (mg)	K-Factor
Organ			
Calves' liver (raw)	73	281	4.0
Hog heart	65	128	2.0
Hog liver (raw)	73	261	3.6
Lamb liver (raw)	52	202	4.0

Seafood

	Sodium (mg)	Potassium (mg)	K-Factor
Fresh or Frozen			
Abalone	70	250	3.6
Bluefish	74	250	3.4
Carp	50	286	6.0
Codfish	105	386	3.8
Croaker	87	234	2.7
Flounder	56	366	6.5
Haddock	61	304	5.0
Halibut	54	449	8.0
Herring	74	420	6.0
Kingfish	83	250	3.0
Lingcod	59	433	7.0
Lobster	60	265	4.0
Mackerel	68	256	4.0
Mullet	81	292	3.6
Perch	79	269	3.4
Pompano	47	191	4.0
Red snapper	67	323	5.0
Salmon	45	399	9.0
Sea bass	68	256	3.8
Sea trout	75	317	4.0
Squid	47	191	4.0
Swordfish	56	366	6.0
Tuna	40	293	7.0

Shellfish

	Sodium (mg)	Potassium (mg)	K-Factor
Shellfish			
Clam (hard)	205	311	1.5
Clam (soft)	36	235	6.0
Mussels	289	315	1.0
Oysters	73	121	1.6
Scallops	255	396	1.6
Shrimp	140	220	1.6

Table 6.1 (continued)

Fresh and Frozen Vegetables and Dried Legumes

Vegetable or Legume	Sodium (mg)	Potassium (mg)	K-Factor
Artichoke, 1	30	301	10
Asparagus	1	183	183
Avocado	21	1,097	52
Bamboo shoots	20	709	35
Beans, dried	7	416	59
Beets, 2 medium	60	335	6
Black-eyed peas	1	303	303
Broccoli, 1 large, fresh or frozen	10	267	27
Brussels sprouts, fresh or frozen	10	273	27
Cabbage, raw	20	233	10
Carrots, 1 large	47	341	7
Cauliflower	13	295	23
Celery, 1 stalk	63	170	3
Chilies, red	9	420	47
Collard greens	43	401	9
Corn, white, frozen	4	226	56
Corn, yellow, fresh	11	219	20
Cow peas	8	229	29
Cucumber	3	80	27
Eggplant	2	214	107
Green beans, fresh or frozen	2	136	68
Kidney beans, dried	3	340	113
Lentils, dried	3	249	83
Lettuce	9	264	29
Lima beans, fresh or frozen	75	478	6
Mung bean spouts	5	223	45
Mushrooms	15	414	27
Mustard greens	32	377	12
Okra	2	174	87
Onions	10	157	16
Parsley	45	727	16

	Sodium (mg)	Potassium (mg)	K-Factor
Vegetable or Legume _(continued)_			
Peas	2	316	158
Pepper, 1 bell	13	213	16
Potato, 1 medium	3	407	136
Radish	18	322	18
Rhubarb	2	148	74
Scallions, 5 medium	5	231	47
Spinach, raw	71	470	7
Squash, average	2	250	125
Sweet potato	22	540	24
Tomato, 1 large	6	488	81
Turnip greens, frozen	12	184	15
Frozen Mixed Vegetables (serving size: 3.5 ounces)			
Broccoli, carrots, and water chestnuts	22	247	11
Broccoli, cauliflower, and red peppers	18	203	18
Broccoli, corn, and red peppers	11	199	18
Carrots, peas, and onions	53	147	3
Cauliflower, green beans, and corn	9	166	18
Green beans, corn, carrots, and onions	10	163	16
Peas, carrots, and onions	60	158	3
Snacks (Recommended Serving Sizes)			
Popcorn and Chips			
Popcorn, unsalted, 1 cup	28	28	1
Potato chips, unsalted, 1 oz. (Lay's)	4	380	95

Table 6.1 (continued)

Snacks (Recommended Serving Sizes) (continued)

	Sodium (mg)	Potassium (mg)	K-Factor
Dried Fruit			
Raisins, ⅔ cup	12	746	62
Figs, 10	1	85	85
Dates, 10	2	541	270
Dried apricots, 10 halves	3	482	160
Nuts and Seeds			
Almonds, unsalted	1	104	104
Almonds, salted (1 oz.)	55	216	4
Brazil nuts, ⅓ cup	1	670	670
Cashews, unsalted, roasted 20–26	8	232	29
Chestnuts, ½ cup	2	410	205
Peanuts, roasted, unsalted (1 oz.)	1	200	200
Pecans, 12 halves	1	63	63
Sunflower seeds	8	258	33

Beverages

	Sodium (mg)	Potassium (mg)	K-Factor
Alcoholic Beverages			
Beer (12 oz.)	18	115	6
Whiskey, gin, rum, vodka, or other hard liquor (1 oz.)	0	1	1
Wine (3½ oz.)	10	116	11
Coffee, Tea, Cereal Beverages (6 ounces)			
Cereal coffee (Postum)	3	97	33
Coffee, brewed	2	117	50
Flavored coffees (average)	25	250	10

	Sodium (mg)	Potassium (mg)	K-Factor
Coffee, Tea, Cereal Beverages (6 ounces) *(continued)*			
Iced tea from mix (sweetened)	13	94	7
Instant coffee	1	72	72
Tea (instant)	1	50	50
Tea (regular)	19	58	3
Carbonated Beverages			
Coca-Cola	14	—	—
Cola	20	7	0.3
Diet Coke	33	—	—
Diet Rite	37	1	0.03
Diet Sprite	45	—	—
Flavored soda	less than 40	about 8	0.2
Ginger Ale	30	5	0.2
Mineral water	less than 5	usually trace	—
Pepsi Light	42	12	0.3
Seven-Up	4	0	—
Tab	27	—	—
Tonic water	2	1	0.5

Desserts

	Sodium (mg)	Potassium (mg)	K-Factor
Dairy Desserts			
Chocolate ice cream	75	240	3
Chocolate ice milk	61	175	3
French custard	84	241	3
Ice cream bar (chocolate coating)	28	107	4
Puddings and Gelatins			
Chocolate pudding, homemade	81	246	3
Gelatin desserts	8	180	22
Rice pineapple pudding	15	55	3

Table 6.1 *(continued)*

Desserts *(continued)*

	Sodium (mg)	Potassium (mg)	K-Factor
Topping (serving size: 3 tablespoons)			
Cherry topping	17	380	22
Chocolate fudge	32	60	2
Chocolate syrup (Hershey)	20	48	2
Cream, half and half, light to heavy, and whipped	18	57	9
Pecans in syrup	—	125	125
Pineapple	17	28	2
Sour cream	36	87	9
Walnuts in syrup	—	88	88
Whipped toppings	9	18	6

Candy

Candy			
Chocolate-covered almonds	17	153	9
Chocolate-covered brazil nuts	13	153	12
Chocolate Kisses (6)	25	115	5
Chocolate with cream center	2	30	15
Gumdrops (28)	10	1	0.1
Hard candy (6)	9	1	0.1
Hershey Dark Chocolate bar	1	97	97
Hershey Golden Almond	17	140	8
Hershey Krackel	49	116	2
Hershey Milk Chocolate	26	119	5
Kit Kat	28	96	3
Lifesavers	3	—	—

	Sodium (mg)	Potassium (mg)	K-Factor
Candy *(continued)*			
Malted Milk Balls	28	113	4
Mr. Goodbar	16	162	10
Nestle Crunch bar	50	110	2

Low-Sodium Salad Dressings and Condiments

	Sodium (mg)	Potassium (mg)	K-Factor
Dressings			
Russian	2	33	16
Thousand Island	2	33	16
Vinegar	2	5	2
Condiments			
Horseradish	17	52	3.0
Homemade sour cream sauce	7	13	2.0
Tabasco sauce (1 teaspoon)	22	3	0.1
Tabasco (6 drops)	15	1	0.1
Perc for natural spices	1.5	22	14.6

7

Keep a Food Diary

Following a low-sodium, high K-factor diet plan will put you more in touch with your body and its relationship to food than ever before. I'm sure you want to begin as quickly as possible. Starting a food diary is the best way to jump right in.

Purchase a small spiral notebook, preferably small enough to fit into a pocket, purse, or briefcase. Record *what* you eat and drink, *how much, when,* and *why.* In addition, at the beginning or end of each day, note your blood pressure and pulse rate. Each evening, evaluate your food in one or two sentences: Was it low sodium, high potassium? Was it balanced? Did you eat enough? Did you eat too much?

Just as each journey—no matter how long—starts with the first step, each life accounts for an enormous amount of food taken one bite at a time. You are now going to make each bite work for you!

HOW THE DIARY WORKS

You will probably discover that low-sodium, high-potassium eating is easy. The advantage of keeping a food diary was vividly illustrated when a colleague at Georgetown Medical School conducted an experiment with some students who wanted to lose weight. The professor introduced me and told the students I was researching food habits and would like each of them to keep a food diary. Each was given a standard spiral notebook in which they listed everything they ate or drank, how much, when, and why. Then each night before retiring, each student spent ten minutes reviewing the foods he'd eaten and wrote a short twenty-five-word summary critiquing his selections.

Every member of that group lost weight. Two years later, the professor who kept in touch with them told me all of them had kept it off. They selected food better than most dietitians would select. They told me that the act of thinking through what they ate forced them to take control, and each recognized what she could do to control her eating habits and still enjoy food. New food habits came to these students almost instinctively.

There is no special way to keep a food diary. Just write what you ate and when, why you chose that food, and whether it was within your low-sodium, high-potassium target. When you take your blood pressure, include the results in your diary—that's the ultimate scorecard.

I have seen people adopt many types of diaries for these or similar objectives. Some people have used commercial daytime planners, others have used elaborate computer recorders. Whatever works is fine. But remember that three things are absolutely essential: honesty, keeping track of everything you eat, and paying attention to the results. Your end-of-the-day critique is the most important step of all. If done correctly, it will give you a better understanding of yourself and your relationship to food. I've noticed that more medical experts have people keep a food diary. This concept can work for you as you seek to improve this aspect of your life.

8

Balance Fat

What do a stick of butter and a bottle of olive oil have in common? They're both fat and provide 9 calories per gram or 252 calories per ounce—or about 85 calories per tablespoon. But olive oil is much better for you than butter.

Most animal fat, for example, butter or the white fat around beef, is solid at room temperature. In contrast, vegetable fat—more specifically vegetable oil—is liquid at room temperature. It's obvious why nutritionists call animal fat "hard fat" and vegetable oil "soft fat."

SATURATED VERSUS UNSATURATED FATS

Saturated and unsaturated fats differ in their chemical structure. The terms *saturated* and *unsaturated* refer specifically to their chemical structure or molecular configuration. Chemists tell us the structure of highly saturated or hard fat is dense and uniform because the molecular linkages holding the carbon atoms together are all used up. In contrast, vegetable oils are not dense and uniform. The linkages holding their carbon atoms together are not used up. The spaces in their molecular structure are open and reactive. When you see "hydrogenated vegetable oil" on a label, it means hydrogen was added to those open spaces, which turns the oil into a solid fat.

Olive oil, a monounsaturated fatty acid (MFA), is an excellent example of an oil that has only one open space. MFA oils are liquid at room temperature, tend to be amber in color, and are somewhat thick or moderately viscous.

Beef lard is a saturated fatty acid (SFA). SFAs are not liquid at room temperature; they are white and hard. This is true of most animal fat.

Sunflower oil is a polyunsaturated fatty acid (PUFA), an oil that has many open spaces. PUFA oils vary in their degree of saturation. The more unsaturated they are, the lighter in color and the more fluid they are. Some are nearly as clear as water.

PUFAs help keep blood pressure normal. In fact, some of these oils can help *reduce* blood pressure. Vegetable oil supplies linoleic acid, a plant oil essential for health. Linoleic acid is the raw material for prostaglandin number 2 (PG2), a substance the body produces. PG2 and other materials produced from it are important in the relaxation and contraction of the muscles that line the arterioles. Therefore, linoleic acid has a metabolic effect that helps to maintain normal blood pressure.

PUFAs also reduce blood pressure by reducing blood viscosity. Remember that reduced viscosity decreases total peripheral resistance to blood flow, and decreased resistance means lower blood pressure.

Saturated fats have a tendency to increase blood pressure by increasing blood viscosity. Increased viscosity contributes to total peripheral resistance, and that increases blood pressure. Obviously, the dietary objective should be to reduce saturated fat; emphasize the unsaturated fat in the diet; and obtain sufficient amounts of a special PUFA, called the omega-3 oils, from fish and vegetable sources. These changes are achieved by shifting emphasis from meat and butter to foods that contain unsaturated fats.

FATS AND CHOLESTEROL

There's another reason to eat more PUFAs and MFAs and fewer SFAs: heart disease. Cholesterol and triglycerides are fats in your blood that your doctor uses as an index to show how clogged your arteries are with fatty deposits. These deposits or plaque, as it is commonly called, consist of cholesterol, among other fats. So, your doctor wants you to maintain both low cholesterol and low triglycerides, since the triglycerides contribute to the plaque as well.

Medical scientists have determined that the lower your blood cholesterol and triglycerides, the less likely your body is depositing plaque on your arterial walls. How high should your cholesterol and triglycerides be? Cholesterol, triglycerides, blood sugar, and many other blood components are expressed as so many milligrams in 100 milliliters of blood. It conveniently allows the use of milligram percent and usually works with whole numbers between 50 and about 300. It is so widely practiced that we often simply use the number. Therefore, it's very likely you'll hear cholesterol expressed as, for example, 180. It really means 180 milligrams percent. (See Table 8.1.)

There are a number of steps you can take to reduce cholesterol. Eat a diet that's low in fat. Avoid or reduce SFAs and use SFAs and MFAs. MFAs, such as olive oil, are ideal for many reasons. Most health professionals recommend that they constitute the major part

Table 8.1		
Cholesterol and Triglyceride Levels		
Age	**Cholesterol (mg %)**	**Triglycerides (mg %)**
Under 50	Less than 180	Less than 100
Over 50	Less than 215	Less than 130

of our fat intake. Total fat intake should not exceed 30 percent of calories; I recommend keeping fat intake at 25 percent of calories. Table 8.2 shows the composition of commonly used fats and oils.

THE PROSTAGLANDINS

There are three prostaglandins. The body doesn't store them, but every cell can make them on demand if the raw materials are present.

Prostaglandins have profound effects on human health. Two have important roles in blood pressure. The first, PG2 (prostaglandin number 2), is made from either of two fatty acids, *linoleic acid* or *arachidonic acid.* Linoleic acid is a polyunsaturated fat obtained

---

Table 8.2

Common Fats and Oils

Oil/Fat	% SFA	% MFA	% PUFA
Butter	68	28	4
Coconut	92	6	2
Corn	13	25	62
Cottonseed	27	18	55
Lard	41	43	16
Olive*	14	77	9
Palm	53	38	9
Peanut	18	48	34
Safflower	9	13	78
Sesame	14	42	44
Shortening	25	68	7
Soft margarine	19	53	28
Soybean	15	25	60
Sunflower	11	21	68

*Considered by most health experts to be the best all-around oil.

from plants, and arachidonic acid, which is converted from linoleic acid by animals, is found in meat. Linoleic acid is designated essential because it is required for the synthesis of arachidonic acid, which is then converted to PG2.

Drugs that inhibit prostaglandin production, such as aspirin or indomethacin, increase blood pressure by increasing total peripheral resistance. This tells a biochemist that PG2, made from linoleic acid, is involved in the dilation of the peripheral arterioles and facilitates blood flow in the kidneys. PG2 also facilitates the release of leukotrienes that help the kidneys remove sodium from the blood. Impaired production of prostaglandin from linoleic acid will very likely contribute to, if not cause, high blood pressure.

Prostaglandins, especially PG2 from linolenic acid, are also important for maintaining good tone of the muscle cells that line the peripheral arterioles. If these muscle cells are too contracted, peripheral resistance increases and blood pressure goes up.

The other important prostaglandin, PG3, is made from eicosapentaenoic acid (EPA). EPA is an omega-3 fatty acid. These polyunsaturated acids are unique because of their detailed structure. EPA is found in the chloroplasts of green plants, but the best source for EPA is blue-skinned cold-water fish, such as mackerel, salmon, and trout.

Unlike PG2, PG3, made from EPA, does not specifically influence peripheral resistance or the kidneys. Ideally a person will eat a diet that provides about three times as much omega-3 oil to omega-6 oil. This will allow the tissues to produce sufficient PG3 to counter the effects of PG2. Since that ratio is difficult to achieve, sensible supplementation with omega-3 oils is recommended. On the other hand, EPA, which produces PG3, does have specific effects on cells. Blood cells and the cells that line the arteries and arterioles absorb EPA and other omega-3 fatty acids, which act as a natural lubricant, facilitating the flow of cells through the vessels and capillaries. In this way, people who have adequate EPA usually have lower blood pressure than people who don't.

The omega-3 oil's effect on high blood pressure might explain in part why vegetarians generally don't have as much high blood pressure as people who eat meat. Although the research is limited, it consistently shows that the rate of high blood pressure is significantly lower among vegetarians, especially vegans, than people who eat meat.

FLAX-OIL AND FISH-OIL SUPPLEMENTS

People with high blood pressure and people who want to maintain their normal blood pressure should be sure their diet contains some linoleic acid and reasonable levels of EPA. That means eating lots of vegetables and fish, especially cold-water fish. People who don't eat fish regularly should either take fish-oil capsules, which contains EPA, or flax-oil supplements, which are a source of alpha linolenic oil (ALA), an omega-3 oil.

I recommend eating about 2 grams of fish-oil daily. This means you must eat cold-water blue-skinned fish about twice weekly, or take three capsules of fish oil daily (excluding cod liver oil). This will provide about 500 milligrams of EPA and a similar level of the similar fatty acid, DHA, or 1 gram daily of these fatty acids.

Some scientists are cautious about fish-oil capsules. They generally base their caution on the high levels of eighteen or more capsules used in clinical studies. Some also point out, erroneously, that these oils contain cholesterol. In the early years, these supplements did; now they don't. At the levels I recommend, these supplements can do a great deal of good and no harm.

ALA is made in the chloroplasts of green plants from linoleic acid. Only plants can make this conversion. Animals, including people, can't make ALA and are dependent on plants for it.

Unfortunately, the diet of most people is just about devoid of ALA because they don't eat sufficient vegetables or range-fed animals (such as rabbits, venison) that accumulate both EPA and ALA. So, the only way we can get ALA is to take a flax oil supplement.

Adding flax oil to your diet, even if you take EPA, will confer an additional benefit by stimulating your metabolism to produce more PG3. Additionally, for those who are vegetarian, it is a completely vegetable oil. Flax oil, which is 52 percent ALA, is a rich golden color and practically tasteless and odorless. It can be purchased in liquid form in bottles, so it can easily be added to your food. Don't fry or bake with it; ALA doesn't tolerate heat well. I personally add one tablespoon of flax oil to my morning bowl of oatmeal or any other cereal. Alternatively, it can be added to salad dressing or used along with vinegar, oil, and spices to make your own vinaigrette. Use it on baked potatoes in place of butter and sour cream. You cannot take too much flax oil, and it will help your program succeed.

Flax oil is also conveniently sold in capsules. Just don't substitute flax oil capsules for EPA completely unless you're a vegetarian. For example, if you take three flax oil capsules or use a tablespoon of liquid flax oil daily, it will equal a 1-gram EPA capsule. This three-to-one requirement is necessary because not all ALA is converted to EPA. Even if you use three tablespoons, or 45 grams, of flax oil (equivalent of three EPA capsules), please take one EPA capsule daily as extra insurance; I recommend this because your metabolism might not convert flax oil to EPA. By the way, reduced heart disease and breast cancer in women are added benefits of using both EPA and flax oil.

In 1982, three distinguished scientists were awarded the Nobel Prize for their work in elucidating the workings of the prostaglandins. Research is continuing on their effects. Someday derivatives of them may help reduce blood pressure in people with impaired prostaglandin production. But for now, food is still the only natural way to obtain sufficient prostaglandins by eating a diet with a variety of vegetables, lots of fish, and natural condiments like garlic and onions.

9

Modulate Sugar Absorption

Chapter 4 introduced the finding that excessive insulin production contributes to high blood pressure by enhancing salt reabsorption. In some people, sugar-rich foods indirectly cause high blood pressure. This means you need to reduce sugar consumption and eat foods that modulate sugar absorption by slowing its entry into the bloodstream.

Most adults consume 130 pounds of sugar per year—that's a heaping (to overflowing) 6-ounce glass full of sugar each day! Though many people will protest that they don't eat that much sugar, surveys have shown that two-thirds of that sugar consumption is hidden in processed foods. For example, an 8-ounce soft drink contains almost seven teaspoons of sugar. Bread, desserts, and fast foods contain sugar. It is everywhere, even in salami, which is loaded with sugar.

COMPLEX AND SIMPLE CARBOHYDRATES

Both complex and some simple carbohydrates are molecularly more complex than simple sugar. Most carbohydrates contain either fructose or glucose, two of the most common simple sugars in nature. Grains or starches, complex carbohydrates, usually contain glucose. Fructose is a simple sugar that makes fruits sweet.

Your body and especially the brain need glucose to function. The problem with eating sugar alone and not part of a complex food, like fruits, vegetables, or grains, is that it crosses the intestinal tract quickly and elevates blood sugar. When you eat candy, or a sugary soft drink, the surge in your blood sugar causes a surge in insulin output, which contributes to sodium retention and elevated blood pressure. The best way to eliminate the problem is to obtain the glucose your brain and body need from simple carbohydrates (fruit) and complex carbohydrates (vegetables, grains, and cereals). The advantage of both complex and simple carbohydrates is that they get broken down slowly in your digestive system and the glucose enters the bloodstream gradually. To be technical, its absorption is modulated. Modulated absorption of glucose or fructose produces a markedly reduced insulin response. And our objective is achieved!

DIETARY FIBER AND BLOOD SUGAR

Fiber, also called roughage, is the indigestible carbohydrate material found in plant foods. Although in a strict sense fiber is not a nutrient because it passes through the system and is not absorbed into the blood, it is one of the most important nutritional components in food. Fiber performs many essential functions on its way through the alimentary canal.

Fiber binds simple sugars. This binding causes the sugars to be released slowly as food moves through the intestinal tract. This modulation in the release of sugar results in a lower insulin output by the pancreas after a meal that is high in sugar. Modulating insulin output is essential to your objective of reducing blood pressure without medication. Fiber does even more; it binds other dietary components such as fat, cholesterol, and even bile acids. All this reduces blood cholesterol. In fact, a high-fiber diet, especially one containing soluble fiber found in fruits, vegetables, and some grains and cereals, lowers blood cholesterol significantly.

The benefits of dietary fiber are discussed in greater detail in the next chapter, along with a table listing the fiber content of common foods.

DIET FOR MODULATING BLOOD SUGAR

Emphasizing foods rich in complex carbohydrates and increasing fiber in your diet can be achieved by eating lots of vegetables, grains, and fruits. Indeed, for most people, this means shifting toward a more vegetarian diet and eating less meat and fewer processed foods.

This emphasis translates into a breakfast that allows many cereals, for example, oatmeal without salt, shredded wheat, or raisin bran. But avoid all sugared ready-to-eat cereals. If your usual breakfast consists of eggs and bacon, you can still have the eggs, just no bacon, and you'll still have room for cereal. The ideal breakfast is cereal with milk and fruit.

Lunch should be light and should consist of vegetables, fruit, and grains. Sandwiches can cause trouble unless the bread is low in sodium and the sandwich contains generous amounts of lettuce, tomato, avocado, and other vegetables. Have fish, vegetables, and a salad with a low-sodium dressing sometimes for lunch.

Dinner affords the widest options. Emphasize vegetables and starches, such as potatoes and rice. Pasta is always good with the correct sauce, for example, tomato, pesto, and even an occasional cream sauce. Include a low-fat protein, such as poultry or fish. Try fruit for dessert.

Obviously, sugary foods and snacks must be eliminated; avoid sugared soft drinks, candy, and sweet rolls. Although there is no direct evidence that sugar substitutes aid weight loss, they are fine here if your objective is to reduce sugar. Artificial sweeteners can serve you well if you like to sweeten your food or enjoy soft drinks. Just don't delude yourself into believing you can eat more food as a reward; rather, see it as a tool to help reduce your insulin production.

10

Increase Dietary Fiber

High blood pressure has many facets to its development; the major ones are excess weight, excess salt, and stress. However, there are secondary factors that don't necessarily cause high blood pressure but clearly contribute to its development and make it worse once it is established. Inadequate dietary fiber consistently shows up as a complicating factor. Indeed, in some studies, simply increasing dietary fiber to over 30 grams reduced blood pressure by a few percent.

Our bodies produce many materials that are eliminated in urine, or by the gallbladder through the intestine itself. Fiber both moves food along the digestive tract and selectively binds waste matter and removes them from the system. It is absolutely essential that the digestive system should have available adequate dietary fiber to bind up these materials and flush them from the body. Generally, this means that each day a person weighing 120 pounds should get 25 grams of dietary fiber, and a person weighing 200 pounds should get 35 grams.

There are about five or six types of fiber, all of which have properties we require. Insoluble or hard fiber, the type found in wheat bran, is the "water carrier" that helps to produce regularity. It produces stool consistency and regularity. As a water carrier, this fiber increases stool bulk and gives it consistency while maintaining softness. Soft but firm stools are important to regularity and the prevention of a number of intestinal problems like appendicitis, diverticulosis, and hemorrhoids. The added water passing through the intestinal tract helps to dissolve and remove unwanted and sometimes toxic materials. This important function helps to reduce the risk of cancer and other illness. Hard fiber is found in all plant food, but mostly in the high-fiber cereals and grains, as well as most vegetables, beans, and tubers such as potatoes. These foods are essential for adequate fiber and the results are obvious whenever a person includes them in their diet.

In contrast to hard fiber, the soluble forms of fiber, such as pectin, gums, saponins, and others, are the best at selective absorption. For example, pectin helps to reduce cholesterol by binding the bile acids produced by our liver from cholesterol and removing them in our stools. Oat bran also removes these materials even better, and guar gum better yet. It also binds the dietary cholesterol and fat and helps to carry them through the system.

FIBER AND WATER

In nutrition, fiber's teammate is water. Water is another nutrient that rarely, if ever, is taken in excess. Because fiber is the plant material that binds water, it can bind you up if you don't get enough water. In the presence of water, fiber makes your stools soft and consistent; in the absence of water, it can make them dry and hard.

The relationship between water and fiber is made clearer by this analogy. Milk contains less water than green peas. The reason you don't eat milk with a fork and drink your peas is because peas have fiber, which gives them their shape and holds the water. You want fiber to do exactly that in your digestive system—give stools consistency without excess firmness.

Fiber cannot perform its cleansing action without water, but our requirement for water extends far beyond that. Indeed, next to air itself, it is the most important of all nutrients. In arthritis, it is especially important for the elimination of waste materials that, in the opinion of some experts, can cause flare-ups. Strive for eight glasses of water daily. Although it is best consumed as pure water, it is okay in other beverages as well.

Sodium in Water

People with high blood pressure should make drinking water a habit, at least four glasses daily. The reason is simply to help facilitate the elimination of sodium. You make the kidneys' work easier.

In addition to drinking more water, you should learn how much sodium is in your water supply. If you live in a hard-water area and have a chemical water softener, you should not drink or cook with the softened water because those softeners remove calcium salts and replace them with sodium. If that is your situation, use bottled water for drinking and cooking. Bottled water, especially mineral water, is excellent. Just read the label to be sure it contains very little sodium. Usually bottled water contains less than 5 milligrams of sodium per 8-ounce glass.

Another option is to use a water purifier that uses reverse osmosis to distill water. These systems are costly, but they produce soft, pure water that is excellent for drinking and cooking.

HOW TO INCREASE DIETARY FIBER

An easy way to get a good start on the fiber you need is to begin each day with high-fiber cereal. Many excellent cereals are available: Fiber One, All-Bran, Bran Buds, bran flakes, corn bran, oat bran, oatmeal, and barley, to name a few. Add unprocessed bran to pancakes or waffles. Eat fruit on cereal, in pancakes, or plain; eat fruit, vegetables, grains, and tubers at each meal. As your fiber intake improves, you'll become more regular.

High-fiber snacks are excellent all day, but drink lots of water. Water increases the value of fiber. Selecting high-fiber cereals for a low-sodium diet plan is difficult. You must read the nutritional table and see how much sodium is provided per serving. If it is 20 milligrams or less, it's okay. If it is over 75 milligrams, be sure it provides at least 10 grams of fiber; if not, it's not worth eating. One cereal that makes the grade is shredded wheat and bran, which is sold by several companies. It provides 8 grams of fiber with no sodium!

A Day with Over 35 Grams of Fiber

Most people have difficulty understanding how 25 to 35 grams of fiber intake daily is achieved, so I've prepared the following table (see Table 10.1). This "day of fiber" exceeds what most people require; for example, a 125-pound woman does fine on 15 to 30 grams daily, while her 200-pound husband needs 35 grams. The woman should use this table as a general guideline, but her husband should stick closely to the plan.

Also recognize that this guide allows for many substitutions. For instance, beans and rice would be an excellent protein entrée that also provides fiber. That combination could easily substitute for a luncheon sandwich.

You cannot get too much dietary fiber. In the past thirty years, I've never observed a study in which people have gotten too much dietary fiber, and that includes one in which volunteers took 90 grams daily.

Table 10.1

A Day of Fiber

Food Item	Soluble	Insoluble	Total	Calories
Breakfast				
Post Shredded Wheat 'N Bran (with ½ cup skim milk)	2.0	6.0	8.0	121
				93
½ grapefruit	0.6	1.1	1.7	39
Snack				
Banana	0.6	1.4	2.0	105
Lunch				
Wheat bread, 2 slices	0.6	2.2	2.8	122
Corn (½ cup)	1.7	2.2	3.9	89
Broccoli	1.6	2.3	3.9	23
Peach	0.6	1.0	1.6	37
Snack				
Apple	0.8	2.0	2.8	81
Dinner				
Brussels sprouts	1.6	2.3	3.9	30
Small salad	1.6	2.2	3.8	50
Potato	0.7	1.0	1.7	200
Melon	0.4	0.6	1.0	130
Snack				
Pear	0.5	2.0	2.5	98
Total	13.3	26.3	38.6	1,218

Table 10.1 (continued)	
A Day of Fiber	
Other Foods Eaten During the Day*	
Food	**Calories**
Fish	200
Sliced turkey	150
Snacks	100
Wine	150
Total calories	600
Total daily calories	1,818

* This day is designed to provide enough fiber, with a little flexibility. There's room to have other desserts or accompaniments, such as wine, up to 1,800 calories for women and 2,200 calories for men.

FIBER SUPPLEMENTS

I'm always asked, "How do I know I'm getting enough fiber?" My answer is: "You should have an easy bowel movement every twenty-four hours. The stools should be well formed, their color should be light brown, and preferably about 10 percent will float."

If your stools don't fit that profile, start using a good fiber supplement.

Metamucil is the standard against which I measure all fiber supplements. It is safe and consistent from one batch to the next. Select the version that is not artificially sweetened; it comes unflavored and orange flavor, either of which is fine. You can take as much Metamucil as you desire. Indeed, it is probably acceptable to take up to six or more tablespoon servings daily. This has been done in many clinical tests.

Drugstores have a wide selection of fiber supplements besides Metamucil. Most of them are made from psyllium seeds, which are mostly mucilage, a type of fiber. They don't contain the seed matrix, are gentle, and also work well. Mix about one or two heaping tea-spoonfuls or one tablespoon with water and drink thirty minutes before a meal. Make sure the one you choose is only a fiber supplement and does not contain any laxative.

Some fiber products contain senna leaf, an intestinal stimulant. Read the ingredients list carefully and avoid anything with senna. Some health food stores sell plant gums, the most common being guar gum, which is also the most effective fiber for lowering cholesterol. However, guar gum should be used carefully because too much will "gum up" the works, actually causing a blockage.

11
Eat More Garlic and Onions

Garlic is a perennial herb and a member of the lily family. Its relatives include onions, chives, leeks, autumn crocus, and lily of the valley, among many others. Garlic, native to Central Asia where it grows wild, has been cultivated all over the world for over five thousand years, making it one of the oldest cultivated plants.

For millennia, garlic has been highly valued in cultures around the world for its culinary and therapeutic virtues. It has been indispensable in Chinese cooking for over four thousand years. In 3000 B.C.E., the Indian healer Charaka, the father of Ayurvedic medicine, said garlic maintains the ability of blood to flow and strengthens the heart. In Egypt, laborers who built the pyramids of Cheops in 2800 B.C.E. were given a daily clove of garlic for strength and protection. Six garlic bulbs were found in Tutankhamen's tomb, which dates from 1300 B.C.E. The garlic was placed there by his priests either to ward off evil spirits or for him to use on his otherworldly journey. Codex Ebers, an Egyptian medical papyrus written in 1550 B.C.E., gives over eight hundred therapeutic formulas, many of which were either based on or used garlic. Over one thousand years later, in

450 B.C.E., Hippocrates ranked garlic as one of the most important of his four hundred "simples," or therapeutic remedies.

Long before processed food, 2 to 5 percent of the people in any society developed high blood pressure. People who develop high blood pressure have minor but perceptible symptoms, with headaches and nosebleeds being the most common. High blood pressure also leads to heart disease, kidney failure, and visual problems. So even though doctors didn't routinely measure blood pressure until this century, people have long recognized the symptoms of high blood pressure. These symptoms were usually called "hot blood." Folk remedies to cure hot blood included garlic.

In the twentieth century, scientists have identified some of garlic's active chemical components, confirming the accuracy of this folklore. In 1921, Dr. Michael Leoper published a paper discussing the blood-pressure-lowering effects of a garlic extract. It not only lowered blood pressure, but it relieved symptoms, such as headaches, dizziness, and occasional nosebleeds. Garlic lowers blood pressure by causing the blood vessel walls to relax and dilate, reducing resistance to blood flow, or peripheral resistance. In 1985, Dr. Ed Block identified *ajoene,* a material in garlic responsible for lowering blood pressure. He confirmed his findings by making the same material in the lab and testing it on people with high blood pressure. His findings have been expanded since then.

Active components in garlic also cause the kidneys to reduce their output of high-blood-pressure-causing hormones. In addition, garlic is a mild diuretic, which causes the kidneys to relax their reabsorption of salt and produce more urine. As they produce more urine, they release more salt, and this reduces blood pressure. Potassium, a second and necessary mineral, is also released, but because garlic supplies potassium, it naturally compensates, to some extent, for potassium loss in urine.

Other researchers in 1921 credited the effects of garlic on intestinal putrefaction. If indeed toxins from intestinal microbes have any role in high blood pressure, garlic could be effective because of its antibacterial properties or because it reduces the absorption of the toxins. The possibility that intestinal microbes can cause high blood pressure is still being researched.

Garlic can further benefit people with high blood pressure by reducing platelet aggregation. When blood components, called platelets, clump together, or aggregate, they form clots, which can cause heart attacks and strokes. Garlic reduces aggregation and helps prevent these internal clots, thus reducing heart attack and stroke risk. This is particularly important for people with high blood pressure because high blood pressure increases platelet aggregation by a large factor.

Garlic can make any dietary program more effective. Its only side effect is a slightly pungent breath. Compared to most modern medications that produce dizzy spells, blackouts, and loss of sexual ability, a little garlic breath doesn't seem so bad.

Onions, aparagus, leeks, and other members of garlic's botanical family all contain some allicin, an active ingredient in garlic and its analogs. They contain these to a lesser extent than does garlic, so they aren't as effective, but they can still contribute to the overall effect. Add chives to the sour cream on your potatoes, put a slice of onion on your salad, and always add a crushed garlic clove to your pot of soup.

GARLIC TABLETS

According to the experts, kyolic garlic, aged garlic pressed into tablets and sold in health-food stores, works as well as garlic. At the first international meeting on garlic, papers were presented to show that aged, kyolic garlic has the same properties as fresh, raw garlic bulbs. There are many garlic tablets sold under many names; some are quite expensive. Because there are no clinical studies on this aspect of garlic tablets, the only advice is to try them and see. However, you should always focus on fresh garlic.

GARLIC DO'S AND DON'TS

Do's

- Add a clove of garlic to each serving of soup.
- Add a clove of garlic to a garden salad.
- Add a clove of garlic to each serving of fish, roast, or fowl.
- Add a half clove of garlic to each serving of spaghetti sauce.

Don'ts

- Avoid garlic salt; it's salt.
- Avoid garlic oil except in a recipe.
- Don't let a day pass without eating some garlic.

12

Be Smart
When Dining Out

Restaurants often serve meals prepared and frozen in central kitchens, salt gets added to many items, and sauces often come from institutional-size cans. In general, the amount of sodium and potassium in restaurant food is simply not known. Nonetheless, you can pick your way through the uncharted minefields of restaurants and cafeteria food without your own personal dietician.

My primary rule of thumb for dining out at any time is *eat natural*. And that's not easy in most restaurants. The following are some generally foolproof guidelines:

- Broiled fish, meat, and fowl with no sauce in natural juices is usually safe. Explain to the waiter. Better still, bring a note for the chef explaining that you are following a strict low-sodium diet; she will work with you.
- Sautéed vegetables are generally safe as long as you emphasize that they need to be low sodium. Many chefs salt frying pans or woks to prevent hot oil from spattering.
- Steamed vegetables, such as broccoli or asparagus, are safe. Avoid accompanying sauces; order dishes without them or have them on the side.

- Potatoes and pasta without a sauce are usually the best complex carbohydrates. Season with olive oil, garlic, spices, or lemon. Purchase nonsodium seasonings such as Mrs. Dash or Vegit and always carry them with you.
- Rice is out; restaurants always add salt to rice so forget it.
- Appetizers are difficult because they usually have sauces. Try shrimp with horseradish, not cocktail sauce. Smoked salmon or trout with plain horseradish is generally safe. Request either a small salad with an oil and vinegar dressing or mushrooms sautéed without salt. Avocado or artichoke is also fine; artichokes go well with oil and vinegar, and avocados can be eaten without any sauce.
- Try fruit for dessert. It would be a rare restaurant, indeed, that did not have a piece of fresh fruit or some berries. They make a fine dessert, and a little whipped cream is okay. But you can take a risk and enjoy a fruit mousse or fruit pie without the crust. The salt is in the crust; the fruit mousse part might be high in calories, but it's usually low in sodium.
- Restaurant bread and rolls simply cannot be eaten because of their salt content. You can learn to get along without them; you'll be thinner for doing so and your blood pressure will be lower.

DO'S AND DON'TS FOR DINING OUT

Do's

- Order fish, chicken, or meat broiled without breading. This includes hamburgers (no cheese) without extenders.
- Eat chicken without skin and do not use any sauces.
- Eat steamed, boiled, or even fried vegetables if they are not canned and salt is not added in the cooking.
- Always eat a salad and two fresh vegetables with lunch. An excellent selection is an ungarnished baked potato. You can

enhance it with sour cream, unsalted (sweet) butter, or unsalted margarine. Better yet, use lemon juice.

- Use avocado for an appetizer or get an artichoke and eat it with oil and vinegar.
- Use vinegar and oil on your salad; no substitutes.
- Eat fresh or canned fruit for dessert if fresh is not available.

Don'ts

- Avoid bread or rolls, not even one slice.
- Avoid cheese, cheese sauces, or cheese on any foods, including salad.
- Don't order sauces or gravy on any foods or foods requiring sauce.
- Don't order foods fried in a batter, such as breaded veal, squid, chicken, or fish.
- Don't order fried foods unless they are fried in oil with no salt added either before or after.
- Avoid pies, cakes, chiffons, mousse, or puddings for dessert.
- Don't use enhancers such as Worcestershire sauce or A-1 sauce.
- Avoid rice; it's always salted.
- Avoid soup.

QUESTIONS TO ASK IN RESTAURANTS

You must learn to ask questions in a restaurant. Don't ever be intimidated; it's your health and your money. Most chefs do not mind the extra request of broiled fish or chicken with no salt. And, if things need spicing and you didn't bring your own, ask for Tabasco sauce; remember, a few drops go a long way.

- May I have the salad with oil and vinegar on the side?
- Can my vegetables be prepared without salt?
- May I have some unsalted french fries?

- Will you make my salad without cheese?
- Can the chef fry or sauté my fish (or mushrooms, and so on) without using salt or monosodium glutamate (MSG)?
- May I have a plain hamburger on the plate without fries if they are salted?
- Do you have any fresh fruit for dessert?

BEVERAGES

Seriously limit alcohol consumption; drink sociably but not excessively. It is best not to take an alcoholic beverage at lunch, but if you must, wine spritzers (wine with soda) are good because a little wine goes a long way. I strongly urge you to restrict yourself to one alcoholic beverage daily—a glass of wine, one mixed drink, or a can of beer.

The best drinks are mineral water with a twist of lemon and iced tea with lemon. Fruit juice is also excellent. Tea or coffee is acceptable. Soft drinks are generally fine, but only in *moderation*; consuming too many will significantly contribute to your daily sodium intake.

AIRLINE FOOD

All domestic and major foreign airlines offer low-sodium meals, but you've got to give them plenty of notice. Call your airline at least twenty-four hours before your flight and explain that you require a low-sodium meal; give them your travel time and flight number.

Be cautious, however; there may be pitfalls in your "low-sodium" meal. For example, you might be served a roll or salad dressing that isn't packaged or a breakfast might contain sausage. Even if you request a low-sodium meal, still apply the do's and don'ts given in this chapter.

One option, which people rarely use on airlines or any commercial travel, is to prepare your own food. The sandwiches I have described are easy to prepare; they're filling and nutritional powerhouses. All they require is the extra effort of purchasing or making low-sodium bread, and every one is better than any airline will serve! In addition, pack an apple or other easily eaten fruit. And you'll still be able to partake of the airline beverage service.

13

Assess Your Weight and Fitness Level

When we're young, our lean body mass is considerable. We are more active, and the level of energy necessary to maintain all that muscle is higher. As we age, our need for muscle mass usually declines, and the energy necessary to keep everything working declines in proportion. The energy we need to keep functioning is called the basal metabolic rate (BMR), and it declines normally with age (more on BMR in the next chapter). If everything remained proportional, our weight would decline as well because our fat content would be maintained at a constant percentage, about 22 percent for women and 18 percent for men.

For example, if you're a man and your lean body mass was 140 pounds at age twenty when you were very active, you simply don't require that same lean body mass at age fifty even if you jog 10 miles weekly. Nor should your percentage of body fat be any different. Let me illustrate with an example as shown in Table 13.1.

Unfortunately, in our society where over 50 percent of adults are overweight, the man in my illustration at age twenty is much more likely to weigh over 175 pounds, and possibly as high as 190 at age forty and more at age sixty. Our lifestyle goes against us. Eating

Table 13.1			
Ideal Man: 15 percent Fat			
Age	**Lean Body Mass**	**% Fat**	**Total Weight**
20	140	15	165
40	135	15	158
60	130	15	153

habits are usually established in the teenage years, and our activity levels drop off as we enter the workforce after school. Therefore, energy expenditure from exercise and work declines while we consume the same food calories or more. We usually consume more calories as we get older; for example, meals and snacks become longer, more regular, and are likely to be enhanced with alcohol or soft drinks. Consequently, people usually gain weight as they get older, and it's very, very rare that their body fat percentage declines. Indeed, percentage of body fat usually increases as people get older.

So, how do you deal with your weight if you've got high blood pressure? First, let's decide whether or not you're overweight.

A PERSONAL WEIGHT ASSESSMENT

Overweight is an overworked term; it implies that there is some arbitrary standard that tells precisely how much you should weigh. If you're an average man, in good shape, you'll have 13 to 15 percent body fat. You likely get some active exercise, some tennis or jogging, for example, and would be able to run a mile in under eight and a half minutes. If you're an average woman in good shape, you'll have 20 to 22 percent body fat. Like the average male, you probably get moderate exercise and can run a mile (or equivalent) in under eight and a half minutes without difficulty.

By comparison, if you were a regular distance runner, I would expect you to come in at 8 or 9 percent body fat and wouldn't be surprised at 6 percent for serious marathoners. If you were a fast-moving tennis player, about 13 percent body fat would be normal for men, 15 percent for women. Percentage of body fat is proportionate to physical need up to a point; fat beyond that percentage is just too much fat. And too much fat imposes stress on your heart, other organs, joints, and in many people causes high blood pressure.

If it's possible for you to have your percentage of body fat precisely determined, by all means have it done, because you can determine very accurately how much weight, if any, you should lose.

The best and most precise method is weighing both in and out of water. It requires sophisticated equipment, however, and can't be done at home, or even in the doctor's office. Actually, you can weigh yourself quite accurately in the water if you are willing to get a spring-type bathroom scale wet and have the use of a pool. All you've got to do is weigh yourself (in bathing suit) on the ground; then take the scale into the pool and do the same thing with as little of you out of the water as possible and after breathing out. Simply duck your head under to read the numbers on the scale and hold as little breath as possible. It's a lot of trouble, but it works. Or get in a swimming pool, curl into a ball, and exhale as you hold your head under water. If you slowly sink, you're probably about right. Sink quickly, and you're better off because you've got even less fat. The more easily you float, the greater your excess fat.

Body measurements are another approach. Stand naked in front of the mirror and observe the following: With feet and knees together facing a mirror, do you see a crack of light above your knees and below your crotch? Can you easily find your hip bones? Turn your side to the mirror and exhale. Are your stomach and abdomen flat and your buttocks firm? If not, start working out regularly.

Tape measure your hip-to-waist ratio. Measure around your hips and waist, and divide the waist measurement by the hip measurement. The ratio for women should be 0.8 or less, for men,

0.9 or less. If the ratio is one or more, you are excessively fat and rapidly developing heart disease. Hold your arm out and grip below the biceps. It should be firm and not droop. If it droops and isn't firm, you need more exercise.

You can actually purchase, or in some places use for a fee, a scale that uses sound waves to estimate your body fat content. The process is simple: You stand on the scale for a few minutes and get your results.

ORIGINS OF EXCESS WEIGHT

Your body evolved to survive in a world of scarcity. When there's excess available, it's very good at storing those extra calories as fat. Fat stores calories efficiently. It conserves 9 calories per gram; that's about 3,500 calories for each pound, and it's pliable at body temperature and requires no water for storage.

Carbohydrates, on the other hand, are solid at room temperature and must be dissolved in water to be used by the body. For every pound of carbohydrate, the body requires at least 3 pounds of water. When a carbohydrate is "hydrated," 1 pound, yielding 1,800 calories, becomes 4 pounds of total weight—that's only 450 calories per pound in contrast to fat at 3,500 calories per pound. Aside from sheer bulk, if calories were stored as carbohydrates, the extra water would elevate blood pressure—one more reason why the body stores its reserve calories as fat.

Excess weight comes from consuming more calories than we burn. But beyond that basic fact, there are several other factors that determine why some people are heavier than others on seemingly the same food intake.

First, some people have a lower basal metabolism than others, and it's lowest in overweight people. Their extra fat acts as an insulator; they don't lose as much heat to the environment, for example. Basal metabolism is the daily calorie expenditure needed to stay alive; the energy you would expend if you stayed in bed all day.

Second, there's the set point theory. This theory says that our brain accepts a level of body fat as "normal" and strives to maintain that level, which becomes a set point. Only by changing this set point can we establish a lower, healthier weight.

Third, or perhaps as part of the first two concepts, the cell size, cell number hypothesis emerged. In this concept, during the first two years of life, the body develops a certain number of cells for fat storage. Some individuals develop more fat cells than others, which makes it easier for them to gain weight.

So, if we combine all these concepts, we can conclude that some people have a naturally low metabolism, or develop a high set point that gives them a certain fat level, or start out in life with an excessive number of fat cells. They may store fat either as lots of small fat cells or as fewer, but larger fat cells. Weight loss is the same no matter what the storage form and no matter what the set point. You've got to burn more calories than you consume and keep doing that for a long time. Exercise is the only thing we know that will produce lean muscle.

Suppose you've got to drop a total of 10 pounds of fat. At 3,500 calories per pound, that means you've got to create a deficit of 35,000 calories. You can consume very few calories, even starve, for a day or two, but you can't do it for a prolonged period. You'll need to establish an average daily caloric intake. If you follow the plan in chapter 14, you'll consume 1,000 to 1,200 calories daily. Well, 2,200 minus 1,000 leaves a daily deficit of 1,200. That means you'll lose 1 pound every three days if you're true to yourself. Or, put another way, it'll take thirty days to lose the 10 pounds.

Weight doesn't come off steadily, though. First, you'll drop some stored carbohydrate and extra fluid, which means a big water loss. In fact, I've seen many people lose 5 percent of their body weight in the first five days. But your body will restore lost carbohydrate and water even while you're still losing weight. People who temporarily regain water and carbohydrate weight often despair because they seem to be gaining, not losing. I assure you, they are losing weight; in the clinic we precisely measure fat loss and it would still be declining. There will be times when you seem to gain weight. But, if you're true to yourself and stick with your program, you can lose 1 to 2 pounds each week over a long period of time and gain a whole new outlook on life.

It is absolutely essential that you do a personal assessment to see if you are fit or fat. Strive to get your body into shape so that your general assessment is realistic. If you need to lose some weight, diet sensibly and maintain your sodium-potassium balance at the same time. Set realistic goals so you know where you're going and how you're getting there.

14

Lose Weight Sensibly

Weight control is absolutely essential for controlling high blood pressure. About 30 percent of all people with high blood pressure can cure themselves by simply losing weight. Each extra pound of fat, though it appears inert, requires about 5 miles of extra blood capillaries. To push blood through all those minuscule passages requires somewhat higher blood pressure.

But a more common cause of high blood pressure in overweight people is excess insulin. Because fat cells are less sensitive to insulin in some overweight people, their bodies produce more insulin, and extra insulin signals the kidneys to increase blood pressure.

Excess weight has nothing in its favor, and young overweight people have a shorter life expectancy because they are at greater risk for heart disease, cancer, and stroke. If the excess weight is complicated by high blood pressure and bad habits like drinking or smoking, the risk of an early death increases and the quality of life declines even more.

BASAL METABOLIC RATE

The basal metabolic rate (BMR) represents the number of calories the body needs daily to maintain temperature, blood flow, and urine production, to breathe, and even to think. A calorie is the amount of energy required to increase the temperature of 1 gram of water 1 degree. Scientists express calories in increments of 1,000, or as kilocalories (*kilo* means "one thousand"). The calories that the body burns or are in food are really kilocalories. However, kilo is dropped and the word *calorie* is capitalized. But remember most of the time you see the word *calorie,* capitalized or not, it usually means kilocalories. Think of BMR as the energy you'd burn if you just lay in bed all day. Interestingly, your brain uses a large block of energy.

You can easily calculate your BMR using a pocket calculator. For example, the following formula has been used to determine the BMR of a five-foot, four-inch, thirty-five-year-old woman weighing 120 pounds.

Basic level:		655
4.36 x weight in pounds	4.36 x 120 =	523.2
4.32 x height in inches	4.32 x 64 =	276.5
Total		1454.7
Subtract 4.7 x age (35)		− 164.5
Calories		1,290.2

BMR is 1,290 calories per day.

The basic level (655) is a factor that applies to all women; it was derived by measuring thousands, if not millions, of women. The factor 4.36 accounts for the calories necessary to keep all your organs working, based on your weight. The next factor (4.32) times height accounts for body surface area and the calories lost to either keep the body warm or cool, as the case may be. The factor 4.7 times age accounts for the decline in BMR as an individual ages.

The formula below has been used to determine the BMR for a six-foot, twenty-six-year-old man who weighs 180 pounds. The basic level for all men is 66 with a weight factor of 6.22 and a height factor of 12.7. The age factor is 6.8.

Basic level:		66.0
6.22 x weight in pounds	6.22 x 180 =	1,119.6
12.7 x height in inches	12.7 x 72 =	914.4
Total	=	2,100.0
Subtract 6.8 x age (26)		− 176.8
Calories		1,923.2

BMR is 1,923 calories per day.

How many calories do you use in a typical day? Table 14.1 below shows how many calories our 120-pound woman and 180-pound man burn up daily at varying levels of activity.

Table 14.1

Daily Calorie Use

Activity Level	Multiplier*	Calories (Woman)	Calories (Man)
Mostly inactive (sedentary, sits most of the day)	1.3	x BMR = 1,677	x BMR = 2,500
Moderately active (exercises three to four times weekly; 30 minutes per session)	1.4	x BMR = 1,806	x BMR = 2,692
Very active (exercises more than four times weekly; 30 to 40 minutes per session)	1.6	x BMR = 2,064	x BMR = 3,077
Exceptionally active (exercises six times weekly; 40 minutes per session)	1.8	x BMR = 2,322	x BMR = 3,461

*The multiplier is derived by extensive research on people who are active to various levels. These are quite accurate if a person is honest about her level of activity.

How would an overweight five-foot, four-inch, thirty-six-year-old woman, who weighs 140 pounds, achieve 125 pounds?

Her BMR is (rounded to the nearest whole number):

$$655 + (4.36 \times 140) + (4.32 \times 64) - (4.7 \times 36) = 1{,}373 \text{ calories}$$

If she is moderately active, her daily calorie use is:

$$1.4 \times \text{BMR} = 1{,}922$$

A 1,000-calorie diet would create a daily deficit of 922 calories. If her target is 125 pounds, her goal is clear:

$$15 \text{ pounds} \times 3{,}500 = 52{,}500 \text{ calories} \div 922 = 57 \text{ days}$$

It would take about two months of a 1,000-calorie daily diet, while maintaining a moderately active life, to achieve her target weight. This is a very realistic objective. When she achieves her 125-pound goal, her eating pattern should fit the following level:

$$\text{BMR: } 655 + (4.36 \times 125) + (4.32 \times 64) - (4.7 \times 36) = 1{,}307 \text{ calories}$$

Maintain a moderately active lifestyle:

$$1.4 \times \text{BMR} = 1{,}830 \text{ calories}$$

If she maintains a modest exercise program and eats sensibly, she will easily maintain 125 pounds. At 1,830 calories, it is difficult even for a dietitian to eat a balanced diet, so it is important to supplement with a multiple vitamin-mineral supplement, calcium, fiber, and—to manage arthritis—EPA and flax oil.

How would a six-foot, thirty-six-year-old man, who weighs 210 pounds, achieve 185 pounds? I meet many men in this predicament. You can usually spot them by their bulging waistlines.

His BMR is (rounded up):

$$66 + (6.22 \times 210) + (12.7 \times 72) - (6.8 \times 36) = 2{,}042$$

If he is moderately active, his daily calorie use is:

$$1.4 \times BMR = 2{,}858.8$$

This man now has a clear target for a healthy weight.

EXERCISE

Exercise is an excellent way to control weight. Exercise burns calories, so it helps get rid of extra pounds. Even at rest a fit body has more muscle, which burns more basal metabolic energy than fat. So a fit person sleeping uses more calories than a fat person does.

A little arithmetic tells you that if you exercise at about 300 calories per day and watch your diet, you'll control about one pound every twelve days. (See chapter 15 for more on exercise and suggested activities.) That means that if you burn an additional 300 calories through exercise daily, five days a week, and cut out an equal number of food calories, you could lose a pound or more every week. So a 10-pound target loss would take ten weeks.

However, if you exercise regularly, your 10-pound target will realistically reduce to 8 pounds because you'll be building muscle and eliminating body fat, and muscle is heavier than fat. Muscle looks better, however, takes up less space, and improves body size and shape.

As the body ages, BMR declines. A twenty-five-year-old expends 14 percent more calories daily than a sixty-five-year-old. But because people tend to become less active as they get older, the difference is probably more like 30 percent. Table 14.2 illustrates this point using a typical woman and man at various ages. Assume both are moderately active people.

	Table 14.2	
	BMR and Age	
Age	**Woman** **(5 ft. 6 in., 130 lbs.)** **Calories**	**Man** **(6 ft., 190 lbs.)** **Calories**
25	1,947	2,789
35	1,889	2,694
45	1,814	2,598
55	1,749	2,503
65	1,683	2,408

DIETING

A recent study of two major nationally franchised diet programs gave some startling results. Of the people who lost over 50 pounds, two years later, less than 10 percent had kept it off. Over 60 percent had gained it back, and about 10 more pounds besides. In fact, the dieters proved the programs work well for weight loss. However, the weight losers proved they have a problem, and that is keeping it off!

Dieting for weight loss is simple in principle: All you've got to do is reduce your caloric intake, carry out a normal routine, get about 200 to 250 calories of exercise, and you've done it.

Start by following some rules that are a proven aid to dieting. These guidelines will also help you develop new eating habits, which will help you keep the weight off. These rules, identified by experts over many years, have been refined by people who have lost weight using them.

Rule 1. Food Diary

Keep an accurate food diary and write a critique of what you ate at the end of each day. Don't omit a single morsel. Record your blood pressure also.

Rule 2. Bulk at Each Meal

Salads, fruits, cereals, grains, and vegetables can be used in unlimited amounts. Every meal should include a vegetable, grain, or salad. Eating bulky low-calorie foods is more satisfying and will slow your eating. Compare a 1-ounce pat of butter, which contains 250 calories, to a head of lettuce or a large apple, which contains about 150 calories. Throw in a large carrot for another 100 calories. You can swallow an ounce of butter in an instant without chewing but not the apple, lettuce, or carrot. That's what bulk is all about.

Rule 3. Avoid Red Meat

Don't eat red meat; eat fish and poultry (skin removed) barbecued or broiled.

Rule 4. Eat Starchy Foods

Eat rice, baked potato (no butter or sour cream), or pasta (plain tomato sauce). Always eat a single serving. Snack on popcorn with no butter or salt.

Rule 5. Eat Green Vegetables

Eat all the green salad you want; snack on raw vegetables.

Rule 6. Fruit for Dessert

If you must eat dessert, make it fresh fruit—an apple, pear, orange, or grapefruit.

Rule 7. Alcohol

No alcoholic beverages!

Rule 8. Purchase a Book That Gives Calories, Sodium, and Potassium

I strongly urge you to obtain *Bowes & Church's Food Values of Portions Commonly Used,* by Jean A. T. Pennington, Anna De Planter Bowes, and Helen Church (Philadelphia: Lippincott, 1998).

Rule 9. Fat Bag

Every time you lose a pound of weight, put a pound of sand in a cloth bag. Put the bag in a prominent place. If you regain a pound, remove it from the bag. Start a new bag every 10 pounds.

Rule 10. K-Factor

Limit each meal to 200 milligrams of sodium; be sure to get 3,000 milligrams of potassium daily. Strive for a K-factor of 3 or more. If in doubt, use a little salt substitute (preferably not potassium chloride) at mealtime.

THE SEVEN-DAY QUICK-LOSS DIET

We put weight on slowly, but we want to get it off quickly. With that in mind, I've devised a plan that works well, doesn't compromise your health, and will take about 5 percent of your weight off in a week to 10 days.

It's simple. One day use a 230-calorie meal substitute (such as Carnation Instant Breakfast) four times (breakfast, lunch, dinner, and snack). Before drinking each meal substitute, take a fiber supplement. The next day, eat one complete meal with fish and two meal substitutes. Don't be tempted to use the meal substitutes every day; it is difficult for one day let alone three or more. When people try that, they usually destroy everything they accomplish within two days of going back to regular food.

I am not an advocate of quick weight-loss programs or gimmick diets. However, this plan will initially take off weight quickly, then switch to a regular, sensible diet and keep the weight loss going.

Remember, you need about 65 grams of protein daily to repair, rebuild, and meet normal body needs; very few extra protein calories are converted to fat.

Low-Calorie Day

Three Times Daily

Carnation Instant Breakfast (or similar product) in nonfat milk or soy beverage.	660 K cal.
20 to 30 minutes before protein drink:	
Take a fiber supplement mixed in water.	None
Total	*660 K cal.*
If you don't take a fiber supplement, eat three vegetable snacks, or one piece of fruit divided in half for two snacks.	200 K cal.
Total	*860 K cal.*

Additional Supplements

Multiple vitamin-mineral: two tablets.
Calcium-magnesium: three tablets for
    600 milligrams of calcium.
Vitamin C: 500 milligrams.
Vitamin E plus selenium: one capsule.
EPA: three capsules.

Low-Calorie Day with Food

Breakfast and Lunch

Two instant meals.   440 K cal.

Snacks

Two vegetable snacks.   200 K cal.

Fiber Supplements (three times a day)

Take a fiber supplement mixed in water   None
before each meal.

Dinner

One light meal: salad with lots of lettuce;   250 K. cal.
grated carrots; and 3½ ounces
(100 grams) broiled or baked fish.

Total   *890 K cal.*

Supplements

Multiple vitamin-mineral: two tablets.
Calcium-magnesium: 600 milligrams total.
Vitamin C: 500 milligrams.
Vitamin E + selenium: 400 I.U. +
    50 micrograms (one capsule).
EPA: three capsules.
Flax oil: one tablespoon in protein mix.

Seven-Day Diet Plan

Day 1
Low-calorie day (three or four meal substitutes).

Day 2
Low-calorie day with food (two protein powder meals,
one light meal).

Day 3
Low-calorie day (same as first day).

Day 4
Moderate-food day (two light meals, one meal substitute).

Day 5
Low-calorie day (same as first day).

Day 6
Low-calorie day with food (same as second day).

Day 7
Moderate-food day (same as fourth day).

It's okay to use low-calorie foods, especially diet soft drinks, but they don't help weight loss. Research has shown that low-calorie foods and low-fat or nonfat foods often have the opposite effect because people think they can eat more. Indeed, studies have shown that the fattest people use the most low-calorie, low-fat foods.

WEIGHT-LOSS PILLS AND HERBS

Basal metabolism holds the secret to losing weight easily. Diets work because basal metabolism usually burns over 1,000 calories. On a low-calorie diet of less than 1,000 calories, you'd lose weight even if you stayed in bed. Rather than decrease caloric intake, some people try to take a shortcut by artificially boosting their metabolic rates through diet pills and other stimulants. Although these diet aids may work in the short term, they are not practical or advisable for long-term use, and some pose serious health consequences.

Following are some common diet aids.

- Smoking elevates metabolism by about 10 percent, and on average, smokers weigh about 10 percent less than nonsmokers. Conversely, smokers who quit usually gain weight even if they don't eat more. However, the adverse effects of smoking far outweigh any metabolic advantage it gives.

- Amphetamines, or "uppers" (drugs that stimulate the nervous system), are still prescribed by some doctors to help people lose and control their weight. Although uppers stimulate the metabolic rate, they are not safe because they're addictive and can cause serious mental health problems, and sooner or later you have to stop taking them.

- The herb ephedra (which provides ephedrine) stimulates metabolism and is also used as a weight-loss aid. However, ephedra doesn't work for everyone, and when it does, the body adjusts; so its effect is transient. Still, ephedrine will speed weight loss in a low-calorie diet; you can use it to get started and then stick with the diet alone.

All these examples simply prove that pills or other quick fixes can't help you maintain a healthy weight. Even if a drug or herb accelerates weight loss, people can't be on either one permanently. Ultimately, you must manage your own caloric intake by controlling what and how much you eat and how much exercise you get.

15

Exercise

A study that proves the influence of exercise on high blood pressure was conducted as follows: People with high blood pressure were divided into two groups. One group, the experimental, did supervised aerobic exercise daily in a one-hour session; the other group, the controls, were told to continue their normal daily routine. People were paired by weight, height, and family background.

Both groups were given precise doses of medication to keep their blood pressure at 120/80. The objective was to monitor any changes in medication requirements. Within a month, the medication requirements disclosed the power of regular exercise. The medication required by the exercise group had declined by 20 percent at the end of four weeks and 30 percent by six weeks. The medication required by the control group had increased by 5 percent during the six-week period.

This confirms what is consistently observed in the population at large: People who exercise regularly have lower blood pressure and are much less likely to develop high blood pressure. Moderate regular exercise improves cardiac output, reduces blood pressure, and increases lean body mass. Many studies have shown that regular exercise, for six or more months, reduces blood pressure by about 9 percent.

Improved cardiac output means the heart pumps more blood with each beat. In other words, regular exercise improves the pumping efficiency of the heart by making it a stronger muscle, just as weight-lifting builds big arm muscles. Now that shouldn't surprise you; after all, the heart is a muscle, and how do you improve the strength and flexibility of any muscle? Exercise, that's how!

Every study confirms that moderate exercise must be done regularly and steadily. Regularly means about five times weekly or more. Moderate means that it has to be vigorous enough and long enough each time to have an effect—you need to sweat a little—but not so vigorous that you are constantly sore or exhausted. That translates to vigorous walking for about forty to fifty minutes daily or jogging twenty to thirty minutes. There are many other forms of exercise that work as well or even better, and we'll explore them as alternatives.

When I say exercise reduces blood pressure by about 9 percent, that's an average. In a recent study reported in the *Journal of the American Medical Association,* the reduction amounted to 13 percent or more in some individuals, but on the average was about 9 percent. You can do some quick arithmetic to see that a 9 percent reduction will take some people from the high blood pressure category (135/95) to the high normal category (123/86). If you combine exercise with the dietary guidelines given in this book, you can considerably improve your chances of keeping your blood pressure down. But you've got to exercise regularly, and it takes time for the results to become apparent.

AEROBIC VERSUS ANAEROBIC EXERCISE

Aerobic means "with air"; *anaerobic* means "without air." Anaerobic exercise is a slight misnomer: you usually, but not always, breathe when you do anaerobic exercise. But, though anaerobic exercise elevates your general metabolism, it doesn't exercise your heart and arteries.

Anaerobic exercise is usually short in duration, even if quite vigorous. Your body performs almost without the need to breathe. For example, swimming under water the length of a forty-foot pool, though vigorous exercise, is definitely anaerobic because the energy used during the swim comes from energy-yielding substances within the body. Running a 100-yard dash is also anaerobic. Although it sounds strange, the runner could conceivably run holding his breath. Other examples of anaerobic exercise are weight-lifting, some track events (shot put, discus throw), and everyday activities like running for the bus.

Walking, running, swimming, and cross-country skiing, when done for at least twenty minutes and up to an hour daily, are all aerobic exercises because they involve prolonged use of the cardiovascular system to move large amounts of oxygen in the blood to the entire body. They tone the entire cardiovascular system.

Anaerobic exercise, in contrast, doesn't rely on prolonged use of the cardiovascular system. Anaerobic exercises should be avoided because they temporarily raise blood pressure and, when done regularly for a long period of time, may keep pressure permanently elevated. You know these types of exercise don't help because they create an oxygen debt that has you gasping for breath when you stop. If you can't do it for at least twenty minutes, then don't do it at all.

Which aerobic exercise is best for you? Most people can take a long brisk walk, jog, cycle, or swim. Nowadays, there are devices available to be used at home or in gyms that simulate just about every type of exercise. Table 15.1 lists aerobic exercises and the minimum exercise times required to tone the cardiovascular system. Exercising for the times given will burn about 300 calories.

The best time of day to exercise is open to debate: Physiology gives the edge to the end of the day and sociology to the beginning of the day. Exercise not only tones the body, it relieves stress and tones the mind. Stress for most people is usually highest at the end of the day, so exercise then helps the mind as much as the muscles.

Table 15.1

Time Required for Exercise

Exercise	Time (Minutes)
Brisk walk	40 to 50 (12 mins./mi.)
Jogging	25 (8 mins./mi.)
Bicycling	25 (13 mph)
Nordic Track or cross-country skiing	25
Rowing machine or rowing a boat with a movable seat	25
Aerobic Rider or stationary bicycle	30
Swimming laps with regular strokes	30 to 50
Stair climber	30

Early morning exercise, however, provides a different advantage. Any time you exercise, your brain produces natural opiates called *endorphins,* which elevate your mood. Although they help you feel better after the day is done, they can also help you start the day with an optimistic outlook.

Sociologists have learned that people who exercise in the morning are less likely to quit their exercise program because most people have more control of the early morning hours before the day's obligations take over. All you have to do is rise earlier and get started. Most studies also have shown that morning exercise makes you more efficient during the day. But whatever time of day you choose, the important thing is to exercise.

No one is so unfit, so overweight, so physically handicapped that she can't exercise. I have had the beautiful experience of seeing women in their early eighties start an exercise program to help their arthritis. My own mother, at eighty-two, mounted a stationary bicycle each day and peddled for twenty minutes. If she could do it, so can you. There's an exercise available to everyone just as there are excuses available to everyone.

- "I don't have time." Baloney! Nothing is as important as your health, but nothing is so easily avoided as changing your habits. You'll just have to get up earlier or stop work earlier. Time can be found if you want it!
- "It's dark and dangerous in the early morning or early evening!" No excuse! The plethora of excellent indoor exercise devices available today that have been tested and proven effective make it possible to never go outside.
- "I'm so out of shape it'll take too long." No excuse. It doesn't take as long to get into shape as it took to get out. Start slowly and work up. Walking thirty minutes at a vigorous pace each day is a good start, and it doesn't even require special shoes, except ones that won't cause blisters. Then, work up to fifty minutes, and you're on your way.

CONSULT YOUR DOCTOR

Before anyone with high blood pressure starts an exercise program, he should get the go-ahead from his physician. Ask your doctor if it's okay for you to start a moderate aerobic exercise program. Explain that you're going to start slowly, for example, a walking program, and work up to something more active. The doctor will explain any restrictions, but it's a rare doctor who will say no to vigorous walking unless your condition is exceptionally serious.

Maximum heart rate is the maximum beats per minute you should achieve for your age. Most doctors won't allow you to achieve this rate during an exercise physical unless they must for some specific technical purpose. You can easily determine your maximum heart rate—just subtract your age from 220, then take 70 percent of that number, and you've got the training heart rate (THR) you should strive for in exercising. An ideal exercise will get your heart rate (pulse) to that figure and maintain it for twenty to thirty minutes.

By exercising for twenty minutes, three or more times weekly, you can achieve a training effect. A training effect stresses the cardiovascular system sufficiently so it responds by slowly building more capacity. In the long run, the heart pumps more efficiently, more capillaries develop, and the muscles around the arteries become stronger. Achieving 70 percent of maximum heart rate for twenty minutes is an optimum combination. Take a typical fifty-three-year-old man: his maximum is 167 (220 − 53), and his THR is 70 percent of 167, or 117. So he should exercise vigorously enough to get his heart beating within 10 percent of his THR; that's from about 110 to 123.

When you start out, stay at the low end. After you've been exercising six to twelve months, go nearer the high end. You should not go more than the THR, unless a physician approves or recommends it. You can stay below 70 percent, however, if you extend the exercise time. For example, twenty minutes of jogging at 70 percent equals about fifty minutes of vigorous walking at 50 percent. You can achieve a training effect by simply putting more time into a lower level of activity.

In contrast, don't try the reverse; that is, exercise at 120 percent or even 130 percent of your THR for less time. In our example, it would mean the fifty-three-year-old man exercised to a heart rate of 140 or 150 for about ten minutes. Not only can such behavior damage your heart, it will actually have a negative effect. Stick with what the experts have proven and you'll succeed.

The THR is an average, and you should probably fall somewhere within that range. Just as humans vary in their appearance, so they vary right down to each of the 50 trillion cells that make up the average 150-pound person, and this variation extends to each person's training needs as well. But on average, if you start an exercise program that your doctor says is okay for you, you should be able to achieve your normal THR after a month or two.

Suppose you start with a resting pulse of about 80 or more. Then you'll reach your THR more quickly and have to be more moderate than others. But as you become more fit, your resting pulse will become lower. Suppose you can't exercise fast enough to get to your THR. For example, you have a heart problem that prohibits it. No problem. The THR is an objective that makes it easier because, if exercise is done at a THR for twenty minutes, three to five times weekly, it achieves the training effect. It's a kind of optimum between time spent and level of activity. You can get the same result at a lower level of activity done for a longer period of time.

For example, suppose you can get about halfway to your THR from your resting pulse. That's okay. Simply do it about two and a half times as long. So, instead of jogging twenty minutes, walk briskly for fifty minutes. It's that simple. I emphasize two and a half times because the trade-off is not direct. A little more time is required at the less vigorous level, but the result is the same.

EXERCISE PROGRAMS

I urge you to start a walking program. Walking is easy, doesn't require anything special beyond good shoes, and you get to see things along the way. Just don't stop and talk! Many other variations of exercise are also excellent. As long as the exercise gets you to your THR, and you can sustain it for twenty minutes or more, it is fine. That opens up many possibilities. See Table 15.1 for a list of suggested exercises. Other possibilities are listed below:

Aerobics (low and high impact)
Skating (ice and roller)
Jazzercise (also called Dancersize)
Tennis (vigorous)
Racquetball
Handball
Water polo
Basketball
Hockey

Notice I've left out golf and weight-lifting and specified that tennis should be vigorous. The reasons for these restrictions illustrate what you're trying to accomplish, and it's worth reviewing again.

Golf is a great way to ruin a walk. You walk a little, stop to plan your next shot, talk, wait for others to hit, and so forth. That's not steady exercise even though it takes the better part of a day. It may be excellent recreation, but it's not the way to obtain a training effect.

Anaerobic exercise, like weight-lifting or short-distance running, may add muscle mass, but it doesn't improve aerobic capacity. That is, it doesn't cause the heart to achieve its THR and remain there for twenty minutes or more. Tennis usually fits this criterion because of so many frequent stops for most amateurs. If, however, you play tennis vigorously for a long time (many sets) and don't stop and talk, it will produce a training effect. One advantage is that you'll get good at one of the world's greatest social games and get in shape as well.

TOTAL EXERCISE

Many beginner joggers and cyclists soon feel the effects of fitness and become dedicated. They often start slowly and before long the runners enter 10K races and the cyclists start with century runs. I've had many pupils do this with fantastic results and I'm proud of them. But when people ask me what I do, I always talk about my total program that starts with simulated cross-country skiing.

Jogging and cycling are excellent for cardiovascular purposes. But have you ever noticed that although joggers and cyclists develop muscular legs, their shoulders and arms are undeveloped. It's because the body adapts. If you jog or cycle, you need large muscle mass in your legs, but not in the shoulders. The same but opposite effect unavoidably occurs in the wheelchair "runner," whose shoulders and arms become very well developed.

This is why I'm a fan of simulated cross-country skiing. The Nordic Track machine exercises both upper and lower body. It uses both arms and legs and consequently requires some time to get co-ordinated. The training effect is excellent, however, and the shoulders, arms, hips, and legs become conditioned at the same time. An added benefit is derived from the twisting effect in cross-country skiing. It comes from moving the left arm and right leg simultaneously, and vice versa. This movement helps reduce the fat pads, or love handles, that so many adults develop around the hips.

In addition to twenty to forty minutes of cross-country skiing, a few other exercises are essential to help improve lean body mass and general conditioning: stretching and toning.

Stretch

Before exercising, some stretching exercises are essential because they help prevent soreness and injury. Stretching the calf muscles and Achilles tendons of the legs is easily accomplished by touching the toes while keeping the feet flat on the ground. A good variation is to cross the feet. Don't bounce up and down in an attempt to get closer to the toes; that can hurt and actually damage your tendons. In another variation, stand facing a wall, about one foot away, and lean forward, bracing yourself with your hands. Stagger your feet and bend the forward knee. Keep the rear leg straight with the foot flat on the floor; you will feel a stretch in the rear leg.

The hamstrings of the upper leg are easily stretched by two methods. While standing, raise one leg about hip high (no higher) and rest your heal on a chair arm or other support; keep your let straight and stretch your arms and try to touch the toes of that foot. Don't bounce; a long slow stretch is best. Alternatively, while sitting on the floor with legs apart face forward, clasp your hands behind your back. Slowly lean forward over your left knee. Try to keep your legs straight. Reverse it leaning over the right knee.

Hip stretches are easily done by kneeling on one knee with your back straight; then lean as far forward as possible over the upright knee. Keep the other knee and foot in position on the floor.

Lower back stretching is essential, especially as people get older. Lie flat on your back, pulling one knee at a time to the chest and holding it for about twenty to thirty seconds. After doing each leg about five to ten times, do both legs together and hold for thirty or more seconds.

If you are up to it, there are daily TV exercise programs that emphasize stretching and limbering. Many of them are quite advanced, and you may not be able to keep up. Just get the motion down properly and go at your own pace. Videotapes of slow-paced exercises are also available.

Tone

Toning exercises tone muscle groups: a flat stomach, thin thighs, hips without love handles, a firm derrière instead of a soft fat one, and tight arm muscles instead of soft hanging flab. Simulated cross-country skiing is good because it exercises the arms, hips, and thighs all at once, but other exercises help tone, too.

Half sit-ups with knees bent will flatten the tummy; but they take time to be effective, so perseverance pays. For women who cannot do a complete sit-up (often the price for pregnancy), there are devices you can purchase that will provide support. One device is a harness you wear that has an elastic band that you attach to a door to assist you in sitting up. Others are laced on a hard mat you lie on, it's hinged with handles at shoulder level that you grip to assist the muscles and make the sit-up easier. In both types of devices, the stomach muscles get toned. Alternatively, get in a sit-up position and simply lift your head as high as possible each time. Slowly it will get easier as your stomach muscles strengthen. Whatever type you do, work up to about thirty daily. You will eventually notice a flattening of your stomach and a reduction in hip circumference.

Love handles are dealt with by holding 10-pound weights (books work well) hip high in front with both hands, feet about twelve inches apart. Rotate slowly as far as possible to each side; hold for about ten seconds. Work up to thirty repetitions on each side daily, and eventually the love handles will disappear. Perseverance is essential.

Thighs are thinned by lying on your side and raising the topmost leg; keep both legs straight; reverse sides and repeat. Start slowly as these can make you stiff and sore, but work up to about twenty repetitions for each leg. Once more, perseverance is required, but results will slowly appear.

Use hand weights to firm arms. You don't have to purchase anything sophisticated; any household object, such as a book or a paperweight, will do. Lift the weight up slowly and bring it down slowly. Remember, the weight need not be heavy, just do the exercise regularly. You can do this while walking or, if you're good, while jogging.

ADDITIONAL BENEFITS

Exercise is synergistic. *Synergism,* from a Greek word, means the sum is greater than its parts. Simply put, if you add the benefits of exercise to your dietary program, you get something even greater than you would have imagined. Satisfaction comes with positive reinforcement. You will begin to find satisfaction as you gain flexibility, burn fat, and develop muscle and discover you can perform tasks you had once thought impossible—such as running 10 miles or bicycling 50 miles.

Physical fitness always improves mental alertness because improved muscle tone improves circulation. Improved circulation brings more oxygen and nourishment to your master organ, the brain.

Sleep will be sounder, but not because you are tired; on the contrary, you will have more energy. You will sleep better because everything about your body is more efficient. Although the restorative power of sound sleep remains a scientific mystery, no one can doubt its miraculous mental and physical value.

Your bowels will function more regularly, another synergistic benefit of exercise with improved diet. Although dietary fiber improves regularity and bowel function, regular exercise, which tones all muscles, including those of the bowel, helps them to respond easily and regularly.

Bones will become larger and denser. Osteoporosis is a decline in bone density due in large part to inadequate dietary calcium and exercise during childhood and adolescence. Once women are past menopause, and men get past the age of fifty, hormonal changes accelerate bone loss, so the problem becomes even more critical. Two factors require personal control: increasing dietary calcium and exercise.

Exercise and Stress

Exercise efficiently relieves stress because it provides a convenient means of eliminating the excess flood of hormones, fats, and blood sugars that spill into the blood from the stress. In stress, the body prepares itself to either stand and fight or to run from the danger. Aerobic exercise after a stressful period will benefit you greatly. That's why I always urge people in high-stress professions to exercise at the end of the day. Since their days are often long, this requires indoor equipment, except during long summer evenings.

Alternatively, many successful people schedule stressful meetings in the morning and use the lunch hour for a twenty- or thirty-minute jog or a long uninterrupted brisk walk. If you can't exercise in the evening or at noon, a morning session still has many benefits. It will condition your cardiovascular system, enabling you to deal more effectively with the stresses of everyday business.

16

Understand and Control Stress

Over the past one hundred years, life expectancy at birth has almost doubled, from the low forties in 1900 to over seventy by 2000. Comparing the most common causes of death in 1900 to 2000 provides insight into what twentieth-century health technology has accomplished.

Communicable diseases were the three most common causes of death in 1900; in 1996, diet and stress-related diseases accounted for the four most common causes (see Table 16.1). Diabetes, suicide, chronic liver disease, and accidents all have dietary and stress connections as well. As the twentieth century came to a close, seven of the top ten causes of death were significantly influenced, if not caused, by stress. Stress is inarguably on the rise, and as stress increases, our health suffers. High blood pressure is caused by stress and is a major factor in heart disease and stroke.

THE RELATIONSHIP BETWEEN STRESS AND DISEASE

Stress causes or influences all the diseases listed in Table 16.1 through its effect on our diet and lifestyle habits. A person who can't control stress in a healthy way may use alternative stress relievers, such as smoking and excessive eating, or may omit beneficial activities, such as exercise. These unhealthy habits can themselves contribute to disease, such as the link between smoking and lung cancer, or high blood pressure and being overweight.

UNDERSTANDING HOW STRESS WORKS

The word *stress* has a personal meaning for each of us. We live in an age of anxiety; just about everyone experiences some level of stress from pressures brought on by a complex, competitive society. Tech-

Table 16.1		
Most Common Causes of Death		
Rank	1900	1996
1	Pneumonia and influenza	Heart disease
2	Tuberculosis	Cancer
3	Diarrhea and enteritis	Stroke
4	Heart disease	Pulmonary diseases
5	Brain hemorrhage (stroke)	Accidents
6	Kidney disease	Pneumonia and influenza
7	Accidents	Diabetes
8	Cancer	AIDS
9	Senility*	Suicide
10	Diphtheria	Chronic liver disease

*Possibly Alzheimer's disease, first diagnosed in 1906.

nically, stress is the actual bodily wear and tear caused by these pressures, or stressors.

Stress isn't necessarily a bad thing. An athlete methodically and purposely stresses her body in training so it will rise to a higher level of performance and the athletic event will not exhaust her. Other examples of using stress to advantage include the practice sessions of police and firefighters, and the everyday exercise many of us do to stay fit. Planned physical stress, such as sensible exercise, can improve our capacity to handle both physical and emotional stress.

To most of us, however, stress means the everyday emotional challenges that take a toll on our health and general well-being. We've all overheard someone comment, "He's getting gray too soon," or "She looks older than her age." Worse yet, when a young person has a heart attack, the comment, "Well, he was under a lot of stress," is often heard.

How we deal with all stress, physical and mental, is based on the fight-or-flight response. This response, which we share with all warm-blooded animals, enables us to avoid or confront physical danger. With the more subtle emotional challenges, however, it can do more harm than good.

The Fight-or-Flight Response

You're walking on a lonely street at night when a man jumps out at you from a doorway. In an instant, you tense up and either start running or stand and fight. The attacker is a clear challenge—technically, a well-defined stressor. Your autonomic nervous system (which doesn't include your brain) puts your body into fight-or-flight mode without any conscious thought on your part. Several very important changes take place in the instant you are confronted by the attacker.

- Digestion stops. This enables your blood to be directed to your muscles, so you can run or fight, and to your brain, so you can think quickly.

- Breathing quickens even before you start running or fighting. This puts more oxygen into your lungs for faster transfer to your blood, so your muscles and brain get more energy.
- Pulse rate quickens, raising blood pressure, which forces more blood to your muscles and brain, delivering extra oxygen that enables energy production.
- Sweating starts instantly. This dissipates body heat caused by the increased blood flow and energy you're about to expend.
- Muscles tense for action, making you ready to run or fight. Tense muscles are better able to withstand physical force, such as a blow or knife wound.
- Clotting chemicals pour into your blood to ensure that bleeding stops quickly if you are injured.
- Energy-yielding blood sugar is released for quick energy, and blood and fat is similarly elevated to provide prolonged energy in case you have to keep running or fighting.

An attack is a clear example of a stressful event—pretty much what a person would have faced eons ago if he encountered a large, wild animal. These physiological processes are part of our genetic makeup.

Physical stress causes your body to produce the hormones norepinephrine (in large quantity) and epinephrine (in modest quantity), which together are called adrenaline. Adrenaline causes the increase in heart rate, blood flow, and blood pressure that enables the fight-or-flight response. Athletes warm up before a contest or workout to get their adrenaline flowing, which prepares their bodies for the upcoming ordeal.

The release of both adrenaline and another hormone, cortisol, is triggered by emotional stress. Cortisol prepares us for vigorous physical activity by releasing reserves of energy substances such as protein, fat, and glycogen held in lean tissue for conversion to glucose as an additional prolonged energy source. Prolonged physical activity burns off the results of this hormonal rush, but in emotionally stressful situations, the blood glucose and fatty acids are not burned off. Generally, we don't leave stressful meetings or family arguments and go have a good workout to burn them off; instead, we might go to a business lunch, have a drink or a cup of coffee, or simply sulk. Each option leaves the body with a serious problem: Elevated blood chemicals that were intended to be dissipated by physical activity. Two insidious by-products of prolonged cortisol elevation are increased stomach acidity and lean tissue breakdown. Therefore, prolonged emotional stress leads to ulcers and a weakened body, causing your muscle strength to actually decline. That's why stress and ulcers seem to go together; ulcers are the result of stress that has no other outlet.

COLONEL SMITH: A TYPICAL EXAMPLE

Imagine an examining room in a Pentagon medical clinic. Air Force Colonel Smith, stripped to the waist, is nearing the end of his annual physical. The phone buzzes and the examining physician takes the call. He hands the phone to Smith: "It's your adjutant, and he says it's urgent."

Smith's adjutant explains to him that a Washington reporter has charged him with misappropriating funds to a major Air Force contractor. The accusations are so serious that they could destroy Smith's career. Smith's stress is of the worst kind: He is trapped and can't do anything about the situation until he returns to his office.

As Smith speaks into the telephone, the doctor sees anxiety, dismay, and fear cross his face. The doctor realizes that Smith is experiencing extreme emotional stress. He grabs a syringe, takes Smith's arm, and extracts a blood sample. After the colonel has been on the phone for fifteen minutes, the doctor gets a second blood sample. He now has three samples: one before the stressful event, one at the beginning of the event, and one after Smith was about fifteen minutes into the stress. The doctor also took blood pressure and pulse simultaneously with an electronic sphygmomanometer.

Smith is a fine physical specimen; six feet, 185 pounds. He maintains excellent condition by running and working out five times weekly. Here's what the doctor found when he examined Smith during the call: Before the call, his resting pulse rate was 56 while sitting. His doctor's first measurement, about five minutes into the call, showed a pulse of about 84; fifteen minutes later, it was almost 100. His blood pressure at rest was 110/70; five minutes into the call, it was 130/85; fifteen minutes into the call, it was 140/95. Blood chemistry at five minutes showed twice the normal levels of adrenaline in his blood. His blood sugar had gone from a norm of 80 milligrams to about 100, and there was a rise in free fatty acids. Fifteen minutes into the call, the adrenaline was more elevated, blood sugar was at 100, free fatty acids were 25 percent above normal, and even his blood cholesterol was 10 percent higher than before the call.

You know from the first chapter that the colonel's kidneys released renin and the renin-angiotensin-aldosterone system went to work. This caused his body to retain sodium and constrict his peripheral arterioles. By increasing peripheral resistance, his brain (the main organ) gets more blood. Higher pulse means more blood flow. Elevated blood sugar provides short-term energy; elevated free fatty acids provide energy for him to go a couple of hours. Increased adrenaline meant that his energy level would remain elevated for hours.

If Smith were going to fly into combat, or run five miles, or engage in some other physical activity, he'd be ready! Instead, all he could do was to have his adjutant pull the appropriate files and notify the correct people of the situation. It would have been best if the colonel could've dropped everything and gone for a run. The run would burn off the extra energy, let the adrenaline stabilize, relax his peripheral arterioles, and return everything, including blood pressure, to normal.

Science tells us that when people are faced with this type of emotional stress regularly, they are more likely to have high blood pressure. Some scientists argue that the increase in blood pressure is the outcome of subtle behavioral changes the person makes under stress. Elevated blood pressure results from a so-called negative adaptation that takes place, which maintains the body in a "ready to fight" state. Overeating, excessive alcohol, and not finding time for exercise are just a few of the possible stress-related behaviors that compound the problem.

The primitive fight-or-flight response is alive and well in the modern environment. Whether you're an office worker, bus driver, or are a night-shift nurse, your body responds to challenges just as it would have ten thousand years ago in a camp attacked by looters. Instead of picking up a spear, throwing a rock, or running and hiding, however, you often must hide your emotions. Though you cover up these stress-triggered biochemical changes, they simmer beneath the surface and take a toll on your health by slowly developing high blood pressure unless you take steps to dissipate their effects and prevent them from happening in the first place.

DEALING WITH STRESS

Whether stress is internal or external, there are things we can do to gain control.

1. Don't try to relieve the frustration caused by stress by creating more stress. Don't drink, snack, smoke, or use chemicals. Tranquilizers will never prevent high blood pressure!
2. Maintain fitness. A conditioned body copes well with stress.
3. Mental conditioning for external stress is equally important. Prepare for the worst eventuality and decide how you would handle it. Once you're ready, what actually occurs will be easy.

17

Change Type A to Type B Behavior

Research has proven that Type A personalities have much higher rates of high blood pressure and, consequently, more heart disease, heart attacks, and strokes than do Type B personalities. Not all Type As have heart attacks, nor do all Type Bs avoid them. In addition, Type A people don't seem to have ulcers, but they are ulcer carriers. Type A people pay a high price for their behavior.

The life of a Type A personality is characterized by high discharges of adrenaline and cortisol. They are likely to also have high levels of cholesterol, blood fat, and blood pressure, as well as high blood levels of the clotting chemicals that increase stroke risk. These risks increase with age, so the sooner you do something about them, the better chance you have of neutralizing them.

Type As are competitive. They have a very hard time listening and preventing themselves from taking control in conversations. They never have enough money, a large enough home, enough friends, or enough anything else for that matter, because they are constantly competing; everything is a score to be beaten.

Type As cannot relax. A vacation with idle time stresses them because they interpret it as time with nothing to do. At social gatherings, they will not only turn a conversation around to the topic they want, they will dominate it as well; or they will eavesdrop, slowly inject themselves into a conversation, and then take it over.

Type Bs are the opposite of all the above. They enjoy recreation and can have fun doing nothing. They are not all wrapped up in their accomplishments and often don't mention them unless asked. They seldom become angry or irritable. Relaxing or pursuing a hobby that kills time does not make them feel guilty.

If you recognize yourself in the description of Type As, compare what you have to lose to what you have to gain by changing your behavior (see Table 17.1). If that is not enough to convince you, think of what it will do for your health. You will:

- Avoid high cholesterol and the need for cholesterol-lowering drugs in the future.
- Avoid high triglycercides.
- Avoid high blood pressure and taking drugs to lower it with all their side effects.
- Avoid high blood sugar.
- Avoid high levels of blood-clotting factors.

About 70 percent of personality is genetic. That genetic base is shaped, changed, and honed by our parents, peer group, and the practical needs to get ahead and earn a living. If you can overcome half that inherited part (35 percent) and change the remaining 30 percent, you can convert about 65 percent of Type A behavior to Type B. This is a pretty healthy blend that should allow you to succeed beyond all but a small percentage of the population and to live long enough to enjoy your success.

Deciding to go from Type A to Type B is only the first step, but it is an important decision you won't regret. Making the change requires focusing on two behavior patterns from which most of the others follow: time urgency and aggressive competitiveness. In Type As, these patterns are compulsive; they do them as automatically as ducking from a flying object.

Table 17.1

Benefits of Changing Type A to Type B Behavior

Change from:	Change to:
Working against unrealistic deadlines.	Setting realistic deadlines that are appropriately competitive.
Impatient with everything, especially with people, including family, friends, and colleagues.	Patient with people, promoting a healthy balance at work and with family and friends.
Defined by work; work is the top priority.	Balance among work, family, and recreation.
Having to dominate, be the authority.	Willing to work cooperatively; confident and deliberate in actions.
Forceful in speech, actions, and human relations.	Comfortable in conversation; learning from others.
Poor listener, only waiting to talk.	Careful listener, persuasive in speech.

DECREASE TIME URGENCY

Time urgency manifests in different ways—finishing other people's sentences during a conversation; feeling fidgety while waiting, even when nothing can be done to speed up the process; arriving early for meetings, flights, and so forth; driving fast, always wanting to "make time"; and an inability to relax and enjoy unstructured time. Decreasing time urgency means managing your time more effectively and working more efficiently. Set goals or priorities by the week or even the month, and use those to determine your daily priorities. Use a calendar rather than a stopwatch.

It is important for Type As to have a daily "to do" list based on the week's priorities. Set time aside each day for the unexpected. If the unexpected doesn't occur, use that time for meditation or other stress-relieving techniques described in chapter 24. Don't use the time to get ahead on other projects unless they're important for concrete reasons, not just those in your own mind.

Screen the outside world. Put the answering machine to work. If you've got a task scheduled and do not want to be disturbed, hang a sign that politely says, "Go away." Stick to your guns, and people will eventually get the message. After all, you'll have to train people to treat you as a Type B; they've only known you as a Type A.

Uncontrollable situations often trigger Type A behavior. When such situations occur, assess your priorities, in writing if possible, and compare them against your goals. Consider these three points:

1. Can anything fail because it was done too well or too slowly?
2. Should you decide when your workday will be finished before it starts?
3. Should you work overtime on your project?

Each question can be usually answered no. You can't control the uncontrollable, but you can control the way you respond. It will be tough at first, but it will slowly become your habit.

BECOME LESS AGGRESSIVE AND COMPETITIVE

The second Type A behavior you'll need to change is aggressive competitiveness. Type A people quickly become hostile and move into a competitive mode. When those feelings start surfacing, use them as your signal to relax. Ask yourself some pertinent questions: "Am I trying to get this person to do something against his basic needs or personality?" "Am I forcing an imaginary deadline?" "Am I becoming angry or anxious because this is not moving fast enough according to my internal deadline?"

Recognize that many people either consciously or subconsciously try to precipitate an argument. So, you must instantly decide if entering the argument has any relevance to your objectives and priorities. In short, will it bring you anything you want or need? If the answer is yes, then you need to figure out how to do it without anger. If the answer is no, shut up. Anger management is discussed further in chapter 18.

We live in a Type A world, and living as a Type B takes courage. In addition, being a Type B is difficult for someone who is naturally a Type A personality. Once you get started, however, you'll find the change is an *autocatalytic process*—that is, it feels so good that it drives itself along.

Now that you have decided to go from Type A to Type B behavior, approach social situations with the objectives you have established here. Use them to listen to others and expand your awareness of Type B people. You will slowly find social situations more interesting and realize there are people all around you who are fascinating and who have accomplished impressive things.

Going from Type A to Type B is like asking people to give money to a worthy cause—most people mistakenly say, "Give 'til it hurts!" but the smart solicitor says, "Give 'til it feels good!"

Tips for Developing Type B Behavior

- Expand your interests outside work.
- Develop friendships with Type B people.
- Take lunch and rest breaks.
- Appreciate things for which you never had time before.
- Revive old traditions or create new ones.
- Establish at least one hobby.
- Always say to yourself, "I deserve to enjoy that."

18

Channel Anger Constructively

Anger is probably the most self-destructive of our emotions and causes severe stress. An angry person with high blood pressure is like a toddler with a hammer—something bad is certain to happen. Preventing and controlling anger is more than important; it is absolutely essential. People who can't control anger almost always have high blood pressure; worse, it often leads to early heart attacks.

Controlling anger is a learned behavior just like any other skill; you must teach yourself to respond differently to upsetting situations. Just as it takes time for a person to learn to become a hothead, it can take years to become skillful at dealing with anger. Although no one method works for everyone, experts offer these tips for keeping frustration from turning into rage.

- Acknowledge you have a problem. Sure, someone else may have set you off, but that doesn't excuse your bad behavior. Next, make an effort to witness your behavior. When you're driving, for example, observe how closely you follow other cars. What do you do that might be angering other people?

Finally, work on modifying your behavior. If driving is what brings out your worst side, work on avoiding tailgating and other aggressive maneuvers.

- Learn new responses to behaviors that previously would have provoked you. Rather than yelling or making obscene gestures at a driver who has cut you off, say, "be my guest," sing, or even make goofy animal noises. This alters your breathing pattern and slows the rush of adrenaline coursing through your body. Then start talking to yourself; say "It's not worth getting worked up over," or "Don't do anything drastic."
- Distract yourself from the frustration. By changing your mental focus, you can temporarily reduce your anger level and possibly keep from doing or saying things you'll regret.

Anger management is essential to life in the modern world. It doesn't mean you need to back down; management means you assert yourself, diffuse the anger, and settle on what is right.

CONTROL NEGATIVE THOUGHTS

People looking for jobs will tell you the heaviest thing in the world is the telephone when you must use it to call potential employers. It is heavy because a job seeker usually projects negative thoughts onto the person she's about to call. Negative thoughts lay the groundwork for anger if the person shows even the slightest tendency to fulfill your negative projection.

A better approach is to prepare for the worst. Write it down if it helps. For instance, "What must I do if . . ."

- He won't take my call.
- She says they have no openings now.

- He says I'm overqualified (or underqualified).
- She says, "Send me a résumé."

If you are prepared, you cannot get angry; you can only say, "I did my best; I'll do better next time," or better still, you will have found an avenue to an opportunity.

HANDLING ACCUSATIONS

Being blamed or accused can be like a boxing match—someone unexpectedly jabs at you and your first impulse is to jab back. However, in the boxing ring the boxers are getting paid to knock each other senseless. When you are accused in the workplace or personal situations, however, you'll be on the employment line, or in jail, or both rather quickly if you start throwing punches. On the other hand, you still need to assert yourself, while creating a win-win situation.

Suppose you were accused (even jokingly) out loud at a party of hitting your spouse. Some people will always be ready to believe the worst. For the sake of your relationships and reputation, you've got to find a way to convince as many people as possible that you don't hit your loved ones.

If you slug your accuser or shout, "It's a lie," these actions won't convince many people; in fact, observers will be more likely to believe the accusation. Instead, you might try putting one of these questions to your accuser: Why would you joke about something so serious? Whoever told you that? Should I dignify that insult, or will you admit you're joking? Who put you up to saying that? Never bring a third party into the situation; in this example, your wife.

Your responses should be built around your own confidence that the truth is with you. You are not defensive, nor are you directly accusing your adversary of lying. And by implying it is a joke, you are offering him a way out of the dilemma he has created for himself.

DAMAGE-LIMITING OPERATIONS

Suppose you're cut off while driving. The best thing to do is to pull to the side of the road or just slow down, collect your thoughts, give the lousy driver a chance to get far away, and resolve to drive more defensively. Examine your relationship with the offending party, and question the amount of power you want them to have over your emotions. Do you really want him to influence your immediate happiness? If so, it's like putting a sign on your car saying, "I'll let any one of you turn me into a raving idiot."

Most anger-producing situations, however, are not so obvious and short-lived as being cut off. Suppose you've been sold a defective product or have been cheated. Your objective is to recover what you can, move on, and avoid similar losses in the future. The techniques you use are called damage-limiting operations, because you've already lost something, and you want to prevent future losses, or limit the damage that's been done.

Anger is positive in such cases. Thank your body for alerting you to the seriousness of the problem and get back in control of the situation by focusing on the future and limiting the damage. And if things don't go your way, learn to let go and get on with your life.

HANDLING ANGER DURING STRESSFUL SITUATIONS

When you are entering a stressful situation that is almost sure to cause anger, your objective is to prevent that anger.

Do say to yourself
- What do I have to do?
- How many ways are there to deal with this?
- There may not be a need to argue. I'll take three deep breaths, collect my thoughts, and relax.
- A sense of humor will be very helpful.

Don't say to yourself
- I have to win.
- I'm going to get angry.
- There is going to be an argument.
- I'm ready for him or them.

In seeking a fair resolution to a confrontation, make an effort to use neutral, nonaccusatory phrases, even if you feel deep inside the need to accuse your adversary.

Do say to yourself and the others
- Let's go at this one point at a time.
- Could we both be right here?
- Could a cooperative effort work? Perhaps we're both right.
- Arguments only lead to arguments. Let's focus on what is right here.
- Let's work together constructively.
- I'm not going to get angry.

Don't say to yourself and the others
- I'm all tensed up.
- This makes me mad.
- You've got it all wrong.
- They are against me.
- She started this argument.
- I'll show him.

If the situation has become very tense, make use of some damage-limiting techniques.

Do say to yourself
- Anger's a good signal; now it's time to get in control and help myself.
- I'm starting to tense up; time to slow down, take a few deep breaths.
- What do I want to get out of this?

- I do not need to prove myself.
- I'll try and contain this.
- What he says may not matter at all.
- There have to be some good parts to this. What are they?

Don't say to yourself
- He can't do that.
- I'll get even.
- I'll not let him get away with that.
- I'll take it right to the top.
- He can't say that to me.
- This will be awful.

Six Steps to Controlling Anger

1. Take deep breaths. Meditate. Practice yoga. Play computer games.

2. Watch your caffeine and alcohol intake. Caffeine promotes anxiety and irritability. Alcohol and drugs can spur you to act out aggressions.

3. Give yourself extra time when doing things; allow for things going wrong.

4. Remind yourself of the impact anger has on your health. Tirades boost blood pressure, trigger premature heart attacks, and lead to ulcers, strokes, and digestive problems. Besides, it never gets you what you want.

5. Don't be so easily offended by another person's actions. Where is it written you can't be cut off on the freeway? Recognize we're all fallible; practice forgiveness.

6. Seek out professional help. Resources include the American Psychological Association, which has an online brochure, "Controlling Anger Before It Controls You."

If the situation doesn't require an instant solution and anger is rising, you might propose a break. This could be the right time to take a breather and return to discuss the issues, one by one, at a later time.

After the situation is resolved, no matter how it turned out, go to a quiet place and reassess what you've been through.

Do say to yourself
- These difficult situations take time to work out. I resolve to try and not take it personally.
- That could have been worse; or, it wasn't as tough as I thought.
- I am definitely making progress.

Don't say to yourself
- Stuff happens.
- He never did see my point.
- That was awful. I should have said more.
- I'll win next time.

19

Control Alcohol

In 1967, a study entitled "The Los Angeles Heart Study" established a clear link between alcohol consumption and high blood pressure. As alcohol consumption increases, so does blood pressure. This unequivocal relationship between long-term alcohol consumption and high blood pressure has been confirmed in study after study. In fact, the Harvard Medical School Health Letter estimates that alcohol consumption accounts for at least 5 percent and possibly as much as 25 percent of high blood pressure!

Now, don't get the idea that everyone who has a cocktail in the evening or a glass of wine at dinner will develop high blood pressure. That's not the point. It's not the occasional drink; it's regular drinking. About four cans of beer, two or more glasses of wine, or three drinks with one ounce of liquor on a daily basis is enough to cause high blood pressure in many individuals. Conversely, the same research indicates that one alcoholic drink daily (one beer, one glass of wine, or one cocktail) will not cause high blood pressure in most people. If you drink moderately, you'll likely have no problem.

CHARLIE'S STORY

After one of my lectures on reducing high blood pressure, I got the following letter about a month later from Charlie, a man in Colorado.

> Dear Dr. Scala:
> I've been following the advice you gave at your lecture in Denver. I've reduced my weight, stopped smoking, and have been taking potassium supplements with no results.

The letter went on to describe that his doctor had prescribed the potassium supplements. Since the doctor's prescription conflicted with what I advise, a call was in order. Boy, did I get a different picture.

Charlie had indeed lost 10 pounds, but at 210 pounds, he was still 35 pounds overweight for his five-foot eleven-inch frame. And he had retained all his bad habits. He faithfully drank three to five ounces of Tennessee sipping whiskey each evening and had sliced beef with gravy for lunch. His doctor, in an effort to follow my program, had prescribed potassium in the belief that if he restored Charlie's K-factor, it would compensate for his poor dietary habits. But he didn't quite get the K-factor message; you don't simply add potassium.

I called the doctor and we set up a simple plan: no more whiskey and a good weight-loss program that followed the dietary rules in this book to restore potassium-sodium balance. Within a week, Charlie's diastolic reading was below 90. Two months later, his weight was down to 195. His blood pressure was still high at 135/85, but he didn't require medication. Charlie also learned something that other regular drinkers don't learn: If he starts the booze again, his blood pressure immediately goes up.

High blood pressure from excessive alcohol is not good; the only way to reverse it is to stop drinking. Drugs that usually work for high blood pressure don't usually work for drinkers. So, the only solution is to "get off the sauce," or at least reduce it to one drink daily.

HOW DOES ALCOHOL AFFECT BLOOD PRESSURE?

Much is known about how alcohol affects the body, but no one is sure how it elevates blood pressure. We can speculate on two possible mechanisms, however.

Some specialists believe that it directly influences the hormones that either elevate or reduce blood pressure. The hormones that elevate blood pressure are overproduced, and the organs don't get the signal to stop. That would explain why medication does not affect alcohol-related high blood pressure. It also explains why blood pressure returns to normal when the booze stops.

Alcohol also alters the potassium-sodium-calcium-magnesium balance in the fluid within and surrounding the cells. This causes constriction of the capillaries with an increase of the peripheral resistance, and high blood pressure follows.

If you're like Charlie, stop drinking! It's that simple. Under any circumstances, if there's even a hint that your elevated blood pressure is alcohol-related, stop!

Try reducing your alcohol intake to no more than a glass of wine or one mixed drink daily. But if your blood pressure remains above normal at that level, you should stop altogether.

Remember, alcohol has negative effects on your body besides high blood pressure. If it's elevating your blood pressure, it's reducing the quality and quantity of your life in many other ways. Only you can do anything about it; and the only thing to do is stop!

20

Avoid Tobacco, Caffeine, and Cocaine

TOBACCO

Tobacco use increases blood pressure. Anyone who smokes makes a big mistake; anyone who has high blood pressure and smokes "squares" the mistake.

Smoking all by itself is a major risk factor for every type of cardiovascular disease (CVD). High blood pressure is also a major risk factor to heart attack and stroke. When you smoke and have high blood pressure, the combined risks for CVD, heart attack, and stroke increase much more than the simple addition of both risks. Indeed, the risk is a multiple of ten. Saying the risk is squared is probably conservative.

CAFFEINE

Caffeine increases central nervous system activity. The pulse rises slightly, and enough caffeine can make a person feel wired. However, caffeine's effect on blood pressure is marginal and doesn't appear to be long lasting. In short, coffee drinking doesn't cause high blood pressure, but if you have high blood pressure, it makes sense to follow the Greek teaching of "moderation in all things."

Caffeine is addictive. If you don't think you're addicted, try to stop drinking coffee for a full week. If you make it for two days, your willpower is sufficiently strong to quit altogether. However, you will likely notice typical withdrawal symptoms: anxiety, headaches, and irritability. These symptoms are similar to those experienced withdrawing from cocaine or heroin; they're just not as strong.

Why not try tea? In contrast to coffee, tea provides the same stimulating effect but has much less caffeine. A cup of tea delivers about 35 milligrams of caffeine. Compare that to about 100 milligrams for a cup of home-brewed coffee, or 150 milligrams for a cup of coffee sold in a coffeehouse. You could have three cups of tea and not reach the same caffeine level you'd get from one cup of home-brewed coffee. Besides, if you're a Type A and want to become a Type B, switching to tea is a great way to start!

COCAINE

If you use cocaine, you're flirting with a heart attack. Cocaine elevates blood pressure. If you've already got high blood pressure, using cocaine and amphetamines is like smoking while standing in a puddle of gasoline. Something very bad is likely to happen.

21

Take a Basic
Daily Supplement

Your body requires nineteen vitamins and minerals daily in addition to protein, fat, carbohydrates, and fiber to function normally. These requirements are expressed in terms of the recommended daily intake (RDI). Vitamins and most minerals are required in trace, or very small, quantities. For example, every day you need just 400 micrograms (400 millionths of a gram) of the B vitamin folic acid. Compared to that, calcium is required in large amounts ranging from 1,000 milligrams (1 gram) for most people up to about age fifty; then the need increases to 1,200 milligrams, and some experts claim 1,500 milligrams is needed. Magnesium's requirement is midway between 200 to 400 milligrams daily. With the exception of calcium and magnesium, all your vitamin and mineral needs can be packed into a single tablet about 1 gram in weight. Taking a balanced multivitamin and mineral supplement daily is insurance against a shortfall.

Use a supplement that provides the vitamins and minerals in the amounts listed in Table 21.1. With the exceptions of calcium and magnesium, supplements that contain values within 10 to 20 percent of those listed in Table 21.1 are readily available in most supermarkets, drugstores, health food stores, and even discount stores. It is important that your supplement contains all these vitamins and minerals and that you take it daily.

Usually the product you select will have less calcium and magnesium than suggested, which I discuss further in chapter 22. Your diet already contains excess phosphorus and about 20 percent of the magnesium you need. If the product you select comes within 20 percent of the calcium, magnesium, and phosphorus levels listed in Table 21.1, it is fine. Don't select a supplement that varies in these three areas by more than that amount.

Most vitamins are safe at ten or more times the RDI, so if you choose to do as I do and take some extra, you don't have to worry—you're not harming yourself. Recent studies of elderly people indicate that our needs increase as we get older, so taking more than the RDI is undoubtedly beneficial. However, taking excessive amounts of some trace minerals, such as zinc, can be detrimental to health, so more is not always better.

COMMON QUESTIONS ABOUT SUPPLEMENT USE

Question: Aren't the excess vitamins and minerals I excreted just creating expensive urine?

Answer: Especially when you're under stress, but even if you're starving, your body will lose some vitamins and minerals daily through excretion. Under most conditions, your urine is truly "expensive." If your blood level of nutrients is high, your urine level will also be high; that is normal human physiology.

Question: Isn't it expensive to take vitamins and minerals?

Answer: In our society, each person spends on average $1 daily on soft drinks. The multiple vitamin and mineral supplement costs less than 25 cents daily. Is your health worth 25 cents a day? Expensive is only meaningful by comparison.

Table 21.1

Recommended Daily Intake (RDI) of Basic Supplements

Vitamins	Amount per Tablet*	Percent U.S. RDI
Vitamin A (as beta carotene)	2,500 IU** (500 mcg RE***)	50.0
Vitamin D	200 IU (5 mcg)	50.0
Vitamin E	15 IU (5 mg alphatocopherol equivalents)	50.0
Vitamin C	30 mg	50.0
Folic acid	0.20 mg	50.0
Thiamin (B₁)	0.75 mg	50.0
Riboflavin (B₂)	0.86 mg	50.0
Niacin	10 mg	50.0
Vitamin B₆	1 mg	50.0
Vitamin B₁₂	3 mcg	50.0
Biotin	0.15 mg (150 mcg)	50.0
Pantothenic acid	5 mg	50.0

Minerals

Minerals	Amount per Tablet*	Percent U.S. RDI
Calcium	125 mg	25.0
Phosphorus	180 mg	40.0
Iodine	75 mcg	50.0
Iron	9 mg	50.0
Magnesium	50 mg	12.5
Copper	1 mg	50.0
Zinc	1 mg	50.0
Selenium	50 mcg	****
Manganese	0.50 mg	****
Chromium	50 mcg	****
Molybdenum	30 mcg	****

   * Two tablets provide 100 percent U.S. RDI for all nutrients except calcium, phosphorus, and magnesium.
   ** International Units.
   *** Microgram retinol equivalents.
   ****U.S. RDI not established.

Question: A salesperson I know sells a brand of vitamins not available in stores. He says they're better and are all natural, but they're quite expensive. Should I use them?

Answer: Just about all vitamins are made by five companies worldwide. Every atom in each vitamin is as natural as the atom in any other vitamin. My advice is to go with a good brand name because brand-name firms have the most to lose if something goes wrong and therefore usually have the best quality control.

Question: I notice some companies have products that are targeted to specific age groups. I can understand supplements made specifically for children, but what about those aimed at seniors?

Answer: If the supplement supplies at least what is listed in Table 21.1, it is fine. A little more won't hurt and can actually help. Some studies have shown that certain age groups, especially older groups, require larger quantities of certain vitamins and minerals.

22

Get Enough Calcium and Magnesium

Calcium and magnesium are minerals that are essential for health. Calcium is needed for strong bones and teeth and for muscle function, nerve function, and more. Therefore, getting sufficient calcium either from foods or food supplements is essential. We require at least 800 milligrams of calcium daily and some health professionals think that we need more. Women, especially, need as much as 1,500 milligrams daily. Calcium is called a *macromineral* because our bodies require a lot. The minimum daily dosage of 800 milligrams of calcium would weigh about 1.5 grams as calcium carbonate or calcium citrate and would be a large pill. In contrast, other minerals, except magnesium, are required in amounts so small they would barely cover the dot in the letter *i*.

Dietary surveys indicate that less than 40 percent of us get the 800 milligrams daily from our diet, let alone 1,500 milligrams. Milk and other dairy products are the major source of calcium. About three glasses of milk daily is equivalent to 800 milligrams of calcium and 1,500 milligrams equals about five glasses. The sodium content of cheese makes it unacceptable on this plan, so the only alternative is deep green vegetables, such as spinach and broccoli. But 800 milligrams of calcium requires about eight stalks of broccoli or about 25 ounces of spinach, both unlikely amounts to be eaten. Most dietary surveys indicate that Americans don't consume nearly enough milk or deep green vegetables to obtain 800 milligrams, let alone the 1,500 milligrams recommended by the government consensus panel. Since calcium is so essential to good health, calcium supplements make good sense. In many cases, they are the only recourse.

Just as the ratio of potassium and sodium is important to each living cell, so is the ratio of calcium outside the cell to calcium inside the cell. Calcium is required by the cell membrane to maintain its integrity. If the ratio of calcium outside the cell to calcium inside the cell drops, because we either don't get enough calcium or we excrete too much, the cell membrane loses its integrity. It becomes "leaky" and allows sodium and more calcium to enter and potassium to leak out. Recent research indicates that excess sodium seems to cause more calcium excretion.

When calcium levels inside the muscle cell become too high, the cell tightens up. Tighter peripheral muscles that line the arterioles means the arterioles and capillaries are more constricted, which increases peripheral resistance to blood flow and blood pressure. The heart has to pump harder to force the blood through the capillaries.

Inadequate calcium can cause the blood pressure to rise. This effect of calcium is indirect, because it's not primary to high blood pressure, but each seemingly minor effect can add up to a major problem.

Water flows smoothly through a garden hose until you either fold it over to stop the flow completely, fold it a little to slow down the flow, or constrict it with a clamping device. Any one of these actions causes the pressure in the hose between the constriction and the faucet to increase. You can even see the hose become swollen, and leaks sometimes spring at weak points.

The garden hose analogy can help us visualize what happens when peripheral resistance increases. Tiny muscles surrounding the arterioles tighten and constrict them. Constricted arterioles restrict blood flow. Restricted blood flow, like the constricted garden hose, means higher blood pressure between the heart and the surface. And the leaks in the hose have their counterparts in blood vessels; the only difference is the damaged item is not easily replaced at the hardware store.

Magnesium is another mineral essential to many bodily functions. It is required for muscle contraction and many processes in metabolism. Nutritionists classify it as a macromineral because we require 400 milligrams daily. Most of our magnesium comes from milk, meat, and vegetables. Surveys indicate that only about 50 percent of people get the correct amount of magnesium daily. In my opinion, nutritionists, dietitians, and doctors don't emphasize the importance of magnesium enough. So the public remains generally uninformed.

Magnesium, like calcium, is necessary for membrane integrity, and integrity of the membrane is essential for maintaining the correct potassium-sodium-calcium ratio. Ultimately, this membrane integrity influences peripheral resistance, because it will cause the muscles to either relax or to remain tense.

Since low blood levels of magnesium have been associated with high blood pressure, a reason other than its membrane effects on the potassium-sodium-calcium system has been sought. There is some evidence to show that renin is elevated when blood levels of magnesium are reduced, and elevated renin produces elevated blood pressure.

HOW MUCH IS ENOUGH?

Unfortunately, no one can give the precise amount of dietary calcium necessary to prevent high blood pressure. That is because potassium, sodium, and magnesium are all involved. Calcium and magnesium work in tandem; magnesium is needed for calcium absorption.

As a general guideline, you need about 800 milligrams of calcium and 400 milligrams of magnesium. If you are a woman before menopause, 1,000 milligrams of calcium is appropriate, and for postmenopausal woman, 1,500 milligrams is better.

It makes sense to use a daily calcium supplement to obtain about 400 to 600 milligrams of calcium as calcium citrate. Ideally, the supplement would also provide about 200 milligrams of magnesium. Many supplements supply this ratio. Some experts, especially health food store proprietors, will say there is a magic ratio of calcium to magnesium, but this is not true. A great deal of research has shown that if you are deficient in magnesium, it affects calcium absorption up to about 200 to 400 milligrams of magnesium daily, depending on your size and activity level. Once you have achieved that required level of magnesium, your body will absorb and utilize its calcium whether you get only 400 milligrams or the 1,200 to 1,500 milligrams recommended.

Food technologists have been able to fortify orange juice with calcium. In fact, a glass of calcium-fortified orange juice provides as much or more calcium than a similar glass of milk. But the orange juice goes one better; it is a potassium powerhouse. Orange juice provides plenty of potassium, is low in sodium, and, with the calcium, cannot be outdone by any other beverage.

23

Take More Vitamin B-Complex, C, and E

Taking a multiple vitamin and mineral supplement, as advised in chapter 20, provides adequate amounts of all nineteen vitamins and minerals. When you live or work in a stressful environment, however, a case can be made for taking more of the B vitamins and vitamins C and E. If you are active and engage in physical activity, more of these nutrients are sometimes required. Review your environment and decide for yourself:

- Do you live under stressful conditions?
- Do you work in a stressful environment?
- Do you commute over thirty minutes in heavy traffic?
- Are you exposed to a smoky or polluted environment?
- Are you exposed to solvent fumes?
- Do you take patented or prescription medication regularly?
- Do you engage in intense physical activity for over thirty minutes daily?

Answering yes to any of these questions could mean you need more B-complex and the antioxidant vitamins, C and E.

B-COMPLEX VITAMINS

All metabolisms require the seven B vitamins. Research has shown that under physical stress, especially physical injury, the body needs more of these nutrients. Similarly, people under emotional stress often feel more relaxed when they take B-complex vitamins in amounts over and above the multiple vitamin and mineral supplement already recommended in chapter 21.

Many experts call the B-complex vitamins stress relievers, and some physicians prescribe them when people are under stress, especially when they feel depressed. Depression and insomnia are stress symptoms. The simplest way to rule out a B-complex shortage is to simply take an extra amount as a daily supplement. If you take a B-complex supplement, make sure your supplement is balanced with respect to the RDI given in Table 23.1.

Table 23.1

The B-Complex Vitamins: Recommended Daily Intake

Vitamin	RD1
Thiamin (B_1)	1.5 mg
Riboflavin (B_2)	1.7 mg
Niacin	1,943 mg
Pyridoxal phosphate (B_6)	2 mg
B_{12}	2 mcg
Biotin	60 mcg
Folic acid	200 mcg

Questions About B-Complex Vitamins

Question: I found a B-complex supplement that claims it is balanced for stress. It contains much more B_6 and very little biotin. Is it better?

Answer: No! There is no stress balance. Those products usually provide large quantities of the inexpensive B vitamins and very little of the expensive (biotin) ones and have absolutely no scientific foundation.

Question: I found a stress formula that provides zinc and magnesium in addition to the B vitamins. Is this a good product for stress?

Answer: Zinc was successfully used to alleviate stress among people who suffered burns to over 40 percent of their bodies. These people were clearly under stress, but their zinc loss was a result of fluid loss.

VITAMIN C

Research suggests that the RDI of vitamin C should be about 100 to 150 milligrams under most conditions. If you live or work in a smoky environment, or must commute long hours in a car while in traffic, you need more vitamin C than provided by the RDI.

When your body is under stress, your vitamin C level drops. Inadequate vitamin C causes leukocytes, or white blood cells, and antibodies to drop below normal levels. These cells drop as much as 25 percent, and those that survive lose as much as 25 percent of their ability to attack foreign agents, which adds up to a 50 percent loss. With this defense against disease weakened, cold viruses can multiply. This explains why a physical stress, like a chill, or emotional stress can bring on a cold. Conversely, vitamin C speeds up the production of antibodies, which is why vitamin C makes the cold less severe.

Physical stress as determined by testing athletes increases the vitamin C requirement. To translate an athlete's need to the average person in a stressful job or a homemaker with several children is not scientifically valid. However, taking up to 1,000 milligrams of vitamin C daily does have some benefits and no negative side effects. A suggested minimum level is between 100 and 500 milligrams of vitamin C daily. These levels can be achieved by starting your day with orange juice and then making sure you get at least four or more servings of fruits and vegetables.

If you decide on a special vitamin C supplement, select one that provides 500 milligrams per tablet. Should you decide you need 1,000 milligrams daily, take one 500 milligrams tablet twice daily, in the morning and evening.

People who regularly use aspirin or other nonsteroidal anti-inflammatory drugs (NSAIDs) require more vitamin C, as do people who use steroids. In both cases, an extra 500 milligrams of vitamin C daily will cover the requirement.

VITAMIN E

Age spots (*fleurs de cimitiere* in French) appear on the backs of our hands, on our faces, and on other parts of the body. Though you can't see them, they also appear on the internal organs.

Age spots are accumulations of pigments involving rancid oils, called *lipofuscin*. French folk wisdom holds that wheat germ or wheat germ oil prevents age spots. The only nutritional way to prevent the onset of age spots is with vitamin E, and wheat germ oil happens to be the best natural source. This folk wisdom goes right to the heart of vitamins E's function: preventing the oxidation of essential oils in the body. In this way, vitamin E actually slows the aging process.

If you want to get 50 milligrams of vitamin E daily, you will need to take a supplement that contains at least 30 milligrams, and you'd be better off taking one that provides 40 milligrams. One advantage of taking extra vitamin E is that your body stores it, unlike vitamin C, which must be replaced daily. Therefore, if you took a 400-I.U. supplement or 240 milligrams once weekly, that would maintain a running average of about 50 milligrams daily if you eat a good diet. Since almost all the most concentrated sources of vitamin E are very high in calories, a vitamin E supplement will more easily fit into your calorie limits.

The vitamin E should be made from D alphatocopherol. It can be in the acetate or succinate form. If it is DL, don't purchase it. The D is the effective form; having both isomers, D and L, can actually reduce the effectiveness of vitamin E.

24

Use Meditation and Biofeedback

MEDITATION

Studies conducted on people before and after beginning a meditation program showed some startling effects. Once their meditation program was well established, their blood pressure dropped, their resting pulse was lower, they slept more soundly, and their cholesterol was lower.

How can that be? Think about everything you've read about stress: it elevates blood pressure, increases pulse rate, elevates cholesterol, and steals sleep. It follows that meditation must relieve stress. Professor Herbert Benson, M.D., of Harvard Medical School, described meditation as the "relaxation response."

There are a variety of meditation methods, but all share the same basic characteristics. Although a teacher is preferable, you can learn meditation on your own.

Set aside a block of time, preferably twenty to thirty minutes, during which you can be completely alone. Early morning or late evening may be best. Find a quiet place where nobody will interrupt you during your allotted time. For people starting meditation, it is best to have a room or even a large closet that is isolated. Some people start by using the attic in their homes. You might even use your car. Adjust your phone so that it doesn't ring; turn on the answering machine. Make certain no radios or TVs are within earshot, or shouting or other loud noises. Meditation is sometimes assisted by white noise. This is not music but noise that becomes a background setting for your meditation that helps you relax. Meditation tapes of background noises such as a quiet surf or rain are often sold in shops and catalogues.

Teachers of meditation usually have students sit on the floor with their back relaxed legs crossed, and hands on knees. Alternatively, some people sit in a soft chair. In any position, your hands should be relaxed and preferably resting on your legs. Teachers usually assign students a mantra to recite over and over. These mantras, which are, as a rule, more sounds than words, become the focus of your attention. You may also focus on a feeling, possibly even visualize a nice scene, such as a mountain lake. Your eyes should be closed throughout this period of reflection.

Anyone who starts meditation learns quickly that two minutes can seem like two hours. Rather than repeatedly opening your eyes to check the time, set a timer that doesn't tick. An electronic, battery-operated timer can be purchased in any hardware store. Start with a five-minute setting and go until it rings. Then increase the time until you are meditating at least fifteen minutes. Once you achieve fifteen minutes, you will begin to notice a change in your ability to deal with stress.

I recommend twenty minutes of quiet time each day. After you have meditated for about fifteen minutes and are relaxed, use the remaining time to reaffirm who you are and what you will become. This self-talk should affirm that you will be optimistic and positive and that you will not allow anger, anxiety, or fear to take over your thoughts.

This is, of course, not all there is to meditation. If you are interested in pursuing meditation further, you can find beginning and intermediate classes in your area.

BIOFEEDBACK

Biofeedback is a method for gaining control of bodily functions normally considered beyond conscious control, such as heartbeat or brain waves. This is accomplished through visualization and the use of a device, such as an oscilloscope, that tells you what your heart rate is. You visualize your heart slowing down or speeding up and the oscilloscope, by recording the heartbeat as waves on a screen, gives you visual feedback that tells you whether you've successfully changed your heart rate. Eventually, through practice, it becomes possible to alter heart rate without relying on the biofeedback provided by the oscilloscope. Simply taking your pulse works well too. Yes, you can actually learn techniques to lower your blood pressure. I don't believe we can control high blood pressure by willpower alone, but if we can bring it down a few points, it is worth the effort because every little bit counts.

The Placebo Effect

We always tell people to ask for the results of a double-blind study when someone makes health claims for herbs, pills, and nostrums. The reason, as you probably know, is to rule out the placebo effect. The placebo effect is an example of the power our brain has over our physiological function. The history of medicine is full of examples of this effect.

People in a clinical study are randomly divided into two general groups: one group gets the real pill or treatment; and the other gets a placebo pill or treatment that cannot be differentiated by any method excepting careful scientific analysis. Then, to complete the double-blind study, the investigators don't know who is getting the real pill and who is getting the placebo.

Careful analysis shows that between about 10 percent for a very clear illness (enlarged prostate) to over 50 percent for a more marginal illness (warts), the placebo effect is about as good as the active material or treatment. Of course, this doesn't hold for something like appendicitis or a broken leg; however, it does for iron deficiency, an inability to urinate from an enlarged prostate, moderate depression, some visual problems, and even precancerous lesions. Indeed, the history of the placebo effect proves that our mind has more power over our health than we generally recognize.

In chapter 1, you learned to take your pulse. Find a quiet place where you can sit in a chair, preferably an armchair, and relax. Take your pulse for a full minute to get an accurate count. Now, close your eyes and concentrate on your heartbeat and try to make it slow down. Do that for a full minute or two and then slowly lift your hand and take your pulse again while consciously trying to make it slow down. Concentrate on each beat.

It takes work. I can usually make my pulse go from about 53 to 48 in less than ten minutes. For me, 48 is about as low as I can get it, on average. If you're willing to work at it, you can achieve similar results. You must get in touch with your body, learn to feel each heartbeat, and concentrate on putting more space between the beats. It works.

Lowering blood pressure by 10 percent is more difficult because you need a device to keep track of it. Sit in a comfortable armchair, put your blood pressure cuff on and measure your blood pressure. After measuring it once, concentrate on slowing each heartbeat, reducing the force of each beat and the pressure between each beat; visualize the blood flowing back into your heart a little more slowly and not being forced out quite as hard. Measure your blood pressure again and, while doing so, concentrate on each beat, the force of each beat, and slowing the flow back into your heart.

I can get my blood pressure down from 110 over 70 to about 105 over 65. In fact, at a recent blood donation I slowed it enough that the only way the nurse could get blood flow was if I did a constant rotational squeeze on the sponge rubber ball. Reducing blood pressure requires visualization and willpower.

25

Use Herbs for Support

No medicine can cure high blood pressure! Medicines can eliminate the symptoms and restore blood pressure to normal as long as you keep taking the medicines. Herbs cannot accomplish this either. If anyone tells you they can, proceed at your own risk of health and money!

Herbs can, however, reduce blood pressure if the high blood pressure has resulted from stress and Type A behavior. Herbs can help reduce the effects of stress.

GINSENG

Ginseng is the only herb known to reduce blood pressure by reducing the anxiety associated with stress, similar to modern tranquilizers. However, it takes time for ginseng to work, so you must use it for two to three weeks to see if it works for you.

Ginseng has been used as a tonic to counteract stress and improve health for millennia. Since its use undoubtedly predates the first Asian medical writings, it is safe to bet that ginseng has been in active use for over twenty-five hundred years. While its actual effects are still elusive to modern medical science, its extensive use over two millenniums suggests it's doing something useful.

In Chinese medicine, ginseng is considered an adaptogen. Since this doesn't fit any standard classification in Western medicine, this term can be confusing. Chinese herbalist physicians say that ginseng is particularly effective for treating a person stressed to his limits. So, its use is appropriate in our complex, competitive, and stressful society.

Western clinical studies of ginseng and its many components have corroborated Chinese claims. Ginseng has many active compounds called genesides, and it is not clear whether ginseng itself or a specific geneside is the active agent. Ginseng has been shown to elicit the following physiological effects:

- Lowers blood pressure.
- Improves reaction to visual and auditory stimuli.
- Improves oxygen utilization during physical exercise.
- Reduces heart rate in physical exercise.
- Improves work output.
- Improves aerobic capacity.
- Improves mood and outlook.

This list suggests that an adaptogen is both a stimulant under some conditions (improves alertness) and a relaxant (lowers blood pressure) under other conditions. Perhaps adaptogen is an appropriate designation given ginseng's ability to adapt to the needs of the user.

In China, Korea, and Japan, ginseng is used in tea. However, in the United States, people usually want a more convenient delivery and want things to work quickly. Hence, ginseng can be found in pills, capsules, and even candies. No proof exists that these forms work or do not work, so experience must be your personal guide.

When using any herb that has a history as rich as ginseng's, it is best to follow traditional use. Ginseng tea is quite pleasant and simply taking your time to drink it will have a calming effect. Take one teaspoon (1.75 grams) dried ginseng root in a cup of boiling water twice daily. Most experts recommend drinking ginseng tea for at least three weeks; others suggest up to three months.

Ginseng is now sold in doses of from 100 to 500 milligrams as tablets, capsules, or powder. It is important to follow the directions that come with these preparations. One consistent point in the folk wisdom surrounding ginseng is that it takes regular use of three weeks to three months for its effectiveness to fully emerge. Therefore, it makes sense to take a smaller dose regularly than a large dose just once or twice.

Although ginseng's history indicates it's very safe for most human use, it makes sense to exercise caution. Common sense dictates that pregnant women should consult their doctors before using any herb or medication, even though ginseng is used by pregnant women in Asia.

VALERIAN

Valerian root was probably the first human tranquilizer, and its appearance in human use is lost in the fog of prehistory. As far as we know, it has been used for at least one thousand years to calm people and help them cope with stress. As with many herbs, it can be found in copies of the *United States Pharmacopoeia* before 1940, and it first appeared around 1850.

Valerian's biochemicals work by attaching themselves to the same sites in the brain that are affected by modern tranquilizers and mood elevators that a doctor would prescribe for stress and anxiety. Valerian use is supported by human clinical and animal research, proving that valerian is effective in helping people cope with stress and the anxiety that follows.

Determining herb dosages can be problematic because herbs aren't standardized as are medications and vitamins. A dose of valerian varies with the method of preparation. Daily use should not exceed 1.5 grams of plant material. That translates to fifteen to twenty drops of a 1:5 tincture in water two or three times daily; 1 teaspoon of root steeped ten minutes in hot water, three times daily; or 1 tablespoon of valerian juice three times daily. Valerian comes with several precautions:

- Not for pregnant women.
- May cause frequent urination.
- Use caution when operating machinery.
- Never use when taking Ativan, Valium, or Xanax. Ask your pharmacist about other drugs.

KAVA-KAVA

Kava-kava, or simply kava, is a muscle relaxant and antianxiety herb that has been clinically tested and proven effective. Kava-kava has been used for hundreds, if not thousands, of years in Polynesia. Since no historical records exist for this area, no one can say when kava-kava's use began, but we do know it has been used as a relaxant for centuries. Clinical studies comparing kava-kava to prescription anti-anxiety medications indicate that kava-kava is reasonably effective.

A daily dose of about 200 milligrams of kava-kava can be spread over three doses of about 65 milligrams each. The actual amount will vary according to the source. Try taking a 40 to 70 milligram dose three times daily and see if it helps you through a period of stress and anxiety.

Kava-kava, like most herbs, has not been tested specifically for safety in either large quantities or in normal use over long periods of time. However, its widespread employment over hundreds of years amounts to millions of human years of use with few reports of side effects. It is a physiologically active relaxant, though, and caution is appropriate when using it, as with any psychoactive medication.

Conclusion

None of the twenty-five steps in this book are beyond any person's ability. Each step is sufficiently easy that there is no reason a person with high blood pressure cannot understand it and make it a part of his daily routine.

Dividends gained by following these steps will eventually find their way into every aspect of life, for you will have faced and defeated an insidious enemy through simple, everyday actions.

Index